prentice-hall
scientific foundations of nursing practice series

Dorothy E. Johnson, Editor

Behavior and Illness
Ruth Wu

Behavior Modification: A Significant Method in Nursing Practice
Michael D. LeBow

scientific foundations of nursing practice series

Behavior Modification

a significant method in nursing practice

Michael D. LeBow
Dartmouth Medical School

prentice-hall, inc.
englewood cliffs, n.j.

Library of Congress Cataloging in Publication Data

LeBOW, MICHAEL D.
Behavior modification.

(Prentice-Hall scientific foundations of nursing practice series)

Bibliography:

1. Nurses and nursing. 2. Behavior modification.
I. Title.

RT42.L37 610.73 72–10297

ISBN 0–13–074179–5

ISBN 0–13–074161–2 (pbk.)

10 9 8 7 6 5 4 3 2 1

Printed in the United States of America

PRENTICE-HALL INTERNATIONAL, INC., London
PRENTICE-HALL OF AUSTRALIA, PTY. LTD., Sydney
PRENTICE-HALL OF CANADA, LTD., Toronto
PRENTICE-HALL OF INDIA PRIVATE LIMITED, New Delhi
PRENTICE-HALL OF JAPAN, INC., Tokyo

Contents

	FOREWORD	*xi*
	PREFACE	*xiii*
one	*SOMETHING IS WRONG WITH THIS PERSON*	*1*
	1.1 Differing Conceptions of Human Problems and a Discussion of Behavior Modification and the Nurse	*1*
	1.2 Behavior Modification	*11*
	1.3 A Synthesis	*21*
two	*SOME OTHER ISSUES CONCERNING BEHAVIOR MODIFICATION*	*24*
	2.1 Formulating the Objectives of a Behavior Modification Program, the Welfare of the Patient, the Human Relationship, Evaluation, and Motivation	*24*
	2.2 A Synthesis	*35*

three *ACCELERATING DESIRABLE BEHAVIOR* 37

3.1 Fundamental Topics 37

3.2 Beneficially Implementing Positive Reinforcement: Types of Reinforcers 49

3.3 Beneficially Implementing Positive Reinforcement: Administering Reinforcers 64

3.4 Beneficially Implementing Positive Reinforcement: Producing Behavior 69

3.5 Beneficially Implementing Positive Reinforcement: Facilitating Meaningfulness and Fostering Prevention by Tapering Off Reinforcement and by Using Social Reinforcers 97

3.6 Beneficially Implementing Positive Reinforcement: Facilitating Meaningfulness and Fostering Prevention by Utilizing Other Helping Agents and Sources of Behavior Modification 107

3.7 Using the Negative Reinforcement Procedure to Accelerate Behavior 124

3.8 A Synthesis 130

four *DECELERATING UNDESIRABLE BEHAVIOR* 135

4.1 A General Statement 135

4.2 Aversive Stimulation 137

4.3 Withdrawal of Positive Reinforcement 142

4.4 Satiation 148

4.5 Extinction 152

4.6 A Comparison of Some of the Deceleration Procedures 158

4.7 *Reinforcing Other Behavior* 162

4.8 *Combining Acceleration and Deceleration Procedures* 165

4.9 *A Synthesis* 171

five DESIGNING AND EVALUATING BEHAVIOR MODIFICATION PROGRAMS 175

5.1 *Introductory Comments and the Importance of Accurate Definitions* 175

5.2 *Precisely Observing and Recording Behavior* 179

5.3 *Some Techniques for Precisely Recording, Clearly Summarizing, and Correctly Evaluating Observations of Behavior* 185

5.4 *Being Skillful in Designing a Behavior Modification Program and Being Critical in Evaluating the Behavior Modification Procedures* 198

5.5 *A Synthesis* 209

six BEHAVIOR PROBLEMS FREQUENTLY ENCOUNTERED BY NURSES 211

6.1 *Apathy* 211

6.2 *Anorexia Nervosa* 213

6.3 *Lack of Self-Sufficiency* 215

6.4 *Social Isolation* 217

6.5 *Objectionable Patterns of Eating* 220

6.6 *Chronic Pain* 222

6.7 *Disruptive Behaviors in the Home* 225

seven *BEHAVIOR MODIFICATION PROGRAMS FOR GROUPS OF INDIVIDUALS* 230

7.1 Token Reinforcement Programs 230

7.2 Community-Based Reinforcement Programs 236

7.3 A Synthesis 242

eight *A CONCLUDING STATEMENT: THE DEVELOPMENT OF SELF-CONTROL* 245

REFERENCES 255

INDEX 265

Foreword

The growth of nursing as a profession and a scientific discipline has been rapid in recent years. New orientations and emphases in nursing education are readily apparent. New organizational patterns to facilitate professional practice are being sought and found. Nursing practice becomes increasingly significant and sophisticated as knowledge is developed along many fronts and is brought to the service of patients. In the face of these changes, and because the knowledge potentially available for practice no longer can be contained within the boundaries of the comprehensive course textbook approach in education, this new approach to the subject matter underlying nursing practice is offered.

The SCIENTIFIC FOUNDATIONS OF NURSING PRACTICE SERIES consists of a number of relatively brief monographs, each dealing with a specific and circumscribed topic. Each monograph is designed to order and integrate pertinent knowledge drawn from widely dispersed sources. Collectively, the series will attempt in time to cover all essential areas, thus providing the fullest scope possible. Such an approach appears to have a number of advantages. The treatment of single topics in separate books permits great flexibility in use in educational programs that vary markedly in the structure and level of courses offered and in the content encompassed or emphasized. It allows the examination of each topic in greater depth than is possible when many issues or concepts must be considered in a comprehensive text, and it encourages consideration of new and emerging foci of interest and development. It avoids the sometimes disjointed nature of publications with multiple authors while simultaneously offering presentation of diverse topics by those especially well qualified to do so. And, finally, it may encourage the development of specialized interest and competence by the advanced practitioner.

The major emphasis in this series is on selected nursing problems. The first concern is for problems that patients are likely to experience in any setting in which nursing is practiced, even though the patients will differ along such dimensions as age; sex; medical diagnosis; and degree, severity, and chronicity of the illness. To the degree made possible by existing knowledge, these problems are described and explained, and the scientific basis for their identification and nursing management is provided. The tentative nature of the basis for prescription in particular will be emphasized, and it is hoped that the presentation will excite in the student or practitioner the skepticism and challenge essential to future contributions to knowledge in the field.

Other volumes in the series cover other aspects of nursing as a field of study and practice. One provides an introduction to the profession and the discipline. Others attempt to synthesize and order knowledge about human behavior in health and illness as a basis for understanding the nature of nursing problems. Still others examine the diagnostic process in nursing, modes of scientific inquiry, and certain treatment methods. Both the underdeveloped nature of nursing knowledge and the steady growth of that knowledge demand that the series remain open-ended, flexible, and subject to early revision.

The scope of nursing practice is broad, and a wide range of knowledge and skills is required among its practitioners. No series of monographs or group of texts can provide adequately for the needs of all students or practitioners in the field. This series is focused upon the needs of baccalaureate and higher degree students but will also serve the needs of many others. The SCIENTIFIC FOUNDATIONS OF NURSING PRACTICE SERIES is an attempt to place in the hands of this group stimulating material of outstanding quality in subject matter and presentation.

Dorothy E. Johnson
Professor of Nursing
University of California
Los Angeles

This book was written for nurses and nursing students who currently are involved with, and who in the near future will direct their attentions to, individuals with behavior problems. The methods espoused in this text have been drawn from the information available in experimental psychology—operant learning in general and behavior modification in particular.

Successful behavior modification programs, that is, programs that result in relevant, effective, and meaningful behavior changes, can be implemented for improving the welfare of both hospitalized and nonhospitalized children, adolescents, and adults. Behavior modification is *not* a circumscribed bag of tricks applicable only in a limited number of situations. Rather, behavior modification is a process, characterized by terms such as "explicit," "precise," and "accurate," that is useful in numerous situations, some of which this book will endeavor to illustrate. The nurse's expanding role as the mediator and designer of behavior modification programs makes adequate preparation in utilizing behavior modification principles necessary. Consequently, the major purpose of this book is to provide this preparation.

Another purpose of this text is to point out the value of teaching patients, their families, and other significant individuals to design behavior modification programs. Behavior modification principles can be used to teach, and behavior modification principles can be taught; both of these activities are discussed in terms of making adaptive behavior changes durable and arming individuals against the unrestrained development of other problems—prevention.

Still another purpose of this book is to dispel the all too frequent belief that behavior modification is dehumanizing. On the contrary, the behavior modification process is a very humane one. Examples will be presented throughout this book that not only illustrate behavior modification practices but also affirm this statement.

The topics that are considered in this text explicate the behavior modification process. Included among these topics are the following: (a) some essential differences between behavior modification and other approaches to patient care as well as some issues that are directly related to employing behavior modification programs; (b) activities that are essential in designing and implementing behavior modification programs; (c) the value of educating the patient and other helping agents; (d) procedures that are useful in accelerating adaptive behavior and decelerating unadaptive behavior (including appropriate combinations of these procedures); (e) procedures that are useful in making adaptive behavior changes durable and extensive; (f) techniques for evaluating what nurses do in behavior modification programs (including both the level of agreement between nurses regarding their observations of behavior and the effectiveness of the procedures that they implement); (g) the applicability of behavior modification principles to groups of people (e.g., mental patients on psychiatric wards); (h) the development of self-control.

The text was planned to avoid inundating the reader with large amounts of new information. Thus, most chapters are divided into sections, with pertinent examples, and are synthesized at the end. Also, subsequent to many of the sections are applications that illuminate the principles discussed. Furthermore, terms and/or questions are provided after each section. These terms and questions should be examined before the material preceding them is read in order to be alerted to the new information, and then they should be defined and answered following this reading.

I wrote this book while teaching at the University of Manitoba. I thank my fellow professors and my students who continually question the behavior modification process and, thereby, stimulate my thinking. In particular, I wish to thank Dr. J. J. Pear for critically reading the entire manuscript and suggesting many valuable changes, and Drs. T. P. Hogan, D. Koulack, and E. Seidman for commenting on early portions of the book.

Furthermore, I am indebted to Albert Belskie, Ken Cashman, and Margaret McNeily of Prentice-Hall for their editorial contributions.

Many praises are owed to Maxine McComas for decoding my (often perplexing) scribbles into a carefully typed manuscript. Similar approbations are owed to Pam Gingera and Anne Greaves for their typing skills.

And last, but not least, I thank Barbara, a deft critic who cares about how much I want to work, and Billy, who joyously is too young to care about such things. Both separately and together, they provide me with much.

M. D. L.

To Six Special People:
Bea and Granddad
Mother and Father
Barbara and Billy

one | Something Is Wrong with This Person

1.1 *DIFFERING CONCEPTIONS OF HUMAN PROBLEMS AND A DISCUSSION OF BEHAVIOR MODIFICATION AND THE NURSE*

Some Introductory Comments about Behavior and This Book

This book is about helping people with behavior problems. Since behaviors are activities, statements about an individual's behaviors describe what he does. For example, statements that a person always reads or that he seldom reads are descriptions of that person's reading behavior. Statements such as "John always frowns," "Bill shouts obscenities at all passers-by," "Susan rarely smiles when she encounters other people," "Betty overeats," or "Tom eats too little," depict what can be termed behavior problems.

In general, society judges that an individual has a behavior problem when he exhibits (1) behavior condemned regardless of how rarely it takes place—a repugnant activity (e.g., incest)—(2) excessive behavior that may not in and of itself be considered repugnant[1] (e.g., laughing or talking), or (3) deficient behavior. When a person engages in a particular behavior too frequently (excessively) in almost all situations (e.g., talking incessantly), or in specific situations (e.g., often talking or laughing during lectures at school), including situations where even one occurrence of that behavior is censured (e.g., laughing when friends relate their difficulties), then society is likely to label the individual's behavior a problem. When a person *rarely* or *never* exhibits a particular activity in situations where society judges it necessary and normal (e.g., rarely or never smiling in the presence of others or rarely or never paying attention to what others say), then society also considers him to have a behavior problem, in this case, a behavior deficiency. Behavior problems need to be altered for the betterment of the individual and society. The terms *problem* and *betterment,* however, are relative and changeable judgments made by the people constituting the society wherein the individual resides. The judgments of some of these people (e.g., psychiatrists) often are more influential than the judgments of the individual himself. This overruling may result in the individual being committed to a treatment he doesn't want (e.g., placement in a mental hospital) for a period of time over which he has little control.

Essentially, behavior problems are relevant activities that society, or more specifically society's "professional labelers" (Ullmann and Krasner, 1969, p. 21), judge as needing change—a change may involve eliminating or reducing the repugnant behavior and the behavior excess or removing the behavior deficiency. The social basis of the designation that a behavior is problematic will be discussed again later in this chapter.

This book is addressed to nurses who work with people afflicted with behavior problems. Thus, nurses in mental hospitals, in community health care centers, in public schools, in general medical and surgical hospitals, in rehabilitation centers for the physically handicapped, in institutions for the retarded, and so on will find the tested procedures discussed in this text applicable to their patients.

As suggested above, when an individual with behavior problems is helped, some of his activities are increased in strength (e.g., the patient interacts more with others), or some of his behaviors are decreased in strength (e.g., the patient stops attacking other patients

[1]There are behaviors (e.g., lying) which most people in society label repugnant but which are tolerated (not considered as behavior problems) until they become excessive.

as often as before, or he entirely stops injuring himself), or both; that is, some behaviors are increased and some are decreased. The powerful procedures necessary to increase and to decrease behavior are sometimes deceptively simple and, therefore, are easily misapplied. Consequently, a major purpose of this book is to explain, to re-explain, to exemplify, and to re-exemplify just how these procedures can best be used.

Decisions about How to Treat Behavior Problems

Treatment experts make assumptions about behavior problems that influence the treatment procedures they implement as well as the goals they formulate for helping individuals with behavior problems. Many psychotherapists, for example, assume that behavior problems are symptomatic of underlying personality problems. In general, these therapists assume that behavior problems are caused by internal events—events inside the person. (For purposes of exposition, this way of thinking will be called the *traditional view.*) Operating on this assumption, the therapists prescribe treatment that attempts to eliminate or somehow to alter the internal state. Krasner (1971) has referred to this strategy of treatment as "evocative-psychotherapy [which is] deducible from a medical, psychoanalytic, or psychodynamic model that aims to alter a person's behavior *indirectly* by first changing intrapsychic organization."[2]

Various schools of psychotherapy espouse different premises and treatment procedures, but many are similar because they focus on assumed causes of behavior problems at levels removed from the behavior itself—they presuppose that the main problem is within the individual.

Behaviorists, in contrast, do not assume that behavior problems reflect internal personality disturbances; so, they do not assume that behavior problems can be remedied only by altering intrapsychic organization. Rather, they assume that behavior problems are learned and—what is becoming less of an assumption and more of an established fact—that such difficulties can be rectified through planned changes in the current external environment of the individual. When carefully planned and systematically executed altera-

---

[2]Leonard Krasner, "The operant approach in behavior therapy," in *Handbook of Psychotherapy and Behavior Change,* eds. A. E. Bergin and S. L. Garfield (New York: John Wiley & Sons, Inc., 1971), p. 614.

tions in an individual's environment are instituted, his behavior problems (i.e., his excesses and deficiencies in specific behaviors or objectionable behaviors per se) can be remedied. The relationship between a behavior and the important environmental events both preceding and following it will be elucidated later in this book. Also, numerous examples will be presented that illustrate the activities of behavior modifiers in changing an individual's current behavior or in producing behaviors that he currently does not engage in at all. The activities of the recipient of behavior modification, as his own treatment expert, also will be exemplified. For now, however, it is important to recognize that essential differences between behavior modifiers and those adhering to a more traditional view exist; that is, the former find it unnecessary to hypothesize that underlying personality disturbances cause behavior problems or, further, that assumed underlying disturbances need to be corrected. The behaviorists conceptualize behavior problems as most closely related to variables outside the person (e.g., variables in the current environment), not inside him. The behaviorist views behavior problems as the major problems needing treatment, that is, behaviors are altered directly not via some underlying personality change.

Proponents of the behavioral and of the more traditional approaches can muster supportive evidence for their respective positions. No attempt will be made to evaluate the vast literature in this area; these assessments can be found elsewhere (e.g., Bergin, 1971; Stuart, 1970). At this point, however, several issues, namely, the symptom, the cause, symptom substitution, and diagnosis will be briefly outlined in an effort to extend the previous discussion and to clarify the behavior modification position.

THE SYMPTOM, THE CAUSE, AND SYMPTOM SUBSTITUTION. The notion that behavior problems are symptoms of deeper ones carries with it the warning that failing to treat the deeper difficulties will result in only *temporary* positive behavior changes or in *supplanting* the old problems with new ones.

Consider, for example, a mental hospital patient who shouts obscenities at all passersby. Many of his behaviors are considered problematic, but shouting obscenities is the most noticeable and the most objectionable to the people with whom he lives.

If this patient's obscenity-shouting is believed representative of an underlying personality malfunction, treatment, according to the traditional approach, should focus on this underlying malfunction.

The behavioral approach to dealing with this patient's obscenity-shouting, however, would involve primarily the behavior problem itself. Thus, a behaviorist would want to know how often the obscenity-shouting occurs, in what situations it is likely to occur, and what reactions the patient receives from others when he engages in this behavior. In other words, instead of asking questions about the presumed underlying disturbance—if in fact there is one, and no one knows for sure that there is—the behaviorist asks questions about the behavior and about the conditions affecting it.

From the behaviorist's point of view, changing the patient's behavior is the most useful approach to helping him conduct himself more capably in society and to helping him lead a more self-satisfying life. The patient acted in ways that resulted in his being labeled disturbed (e.g., he undressed in public, sulked for days, refused to eat, shouted obscenities, attempted to take his own life); it is the *reduction* of these maladaptive behaviors and the *acquisition* of adaptive behaviors that will allow the patient to return to society. In other words, the behaviorist focuses on behavior. For him, effective treatment directly deals with the behavior problem.

Those accepting the traditional view, however, can object to the behaviorist's approach on the grounds that treating the patient's behaviors per se will eventuate in symptom reoccurrence or symptom substitution because the underlying deeper disturbance has been untreated. But the behaviorist maintains that no evidence for the symptom substitution hypothesis can be found (Yates, 1958). He also maintains that if new unwanted behaviors occur after treatment or if previously treated behaviors reoccur, it is due to either ineffective or to incomplete treatment, or simply that treated individuals encounter stresses again and can develop problems once more (Ullmann and Krasner, 1965). According to the behavioral view, therefore, symptom substitution is *not* an automatic by-product of directing treatment toward behavior. Rather, what appears to be symptom substitution—the development of unwanted behavior—can arise because of these other reasons. In Chapter 4, it will be pointed out that one way to reduce the likelihood that new unwanted behavior will replace eliminated behaviors is to provide the patient with adaptive behaviors at the same time as you're attempting to eliminate unadaptive ones.

DIAGNOSIS AND SOME PROBLEMS ARISING FROM LABELING THE INDIVIDUAL. Diagnosis or assessment, as it is traditionally carried out for describing and classifying people with behavior problems, has several difficulties associated with it. First, a diagnostic label is assigned to patients who display certain signs and symptoms; all those individuals who behave in the listed ways receive the same label. But this procedure can be inexact because all the individuals diagnosed the same do not necessarily conform to the textbook description and often engage in other behaviors not described by the diagnosis. In other words, an individual with behavior problems may be placed in a category that reflects some of his behavior problems but that ignores many others. If two individuals are alike in several ways but are different in other important ways, it is unwise to lump them together into one category, unless their similarities have an overriding effect on their other behaviors. Two individuals, both placed in a mental hospital and both given the same diagnosis (e.g., paranoid schizophrenic), may not respond to the same treatment in the same way. They actually may not have the same behavior problems.

Second, a fundamental difficulty is that the diagnosis often is not related closely to the type of treatment offered, possibly because many specific approaches are unavailable. You diagnose to treat. Diagnosis in physical medicine has a closer relationship to the type of treatment eventually administered than does the usual diagnostic practice for patients with behavior disorders. Also, diagnosis, as it is usually carried out for individuals with behavior problems, does not seem to depict accurately the outcome of any method (Stuart, 1970).

Third, increasing evidence shows that assessment devices and measures (e.g., psychological tests, ratings by trained judges who see the same patient) used to arrive at a diagnosis are not very reliable. For example, judges who rate a patient in reference to a specific diagnostic category do not often agree on the classification they assign unless it is very broad (e.g., neurotic or psychotic); finer distinctions, such as paranoid schizophrenic or simple schizophrenic, are very difficult to make (Stuart, 1970).

Fourth, the diagnostic labels assigned to patients may have undesirable effects on them. This result leads to the most important objection to using the traditional categories for patients with behavior problems. Labeling a patient, saying that he is schizophrenic, for example, may markedly alter his relationships with other people, the opportunities he has in his community, and his perceptions about himself. Stuart (1970), has documented evidence of these effects.

The behaviorist also assesses behavior problems. But he concerns himself less with labeling an individual than with ascertaining the relationship of his particular behavior problems to the environment and with delineating the behaviors he must be taught to enable him to be able to live more capably. (The behavior modification approach to assessment of behavior problems will be detailed in Chapter 5.)

Behavior Modification and the Nurse

The environment of the patient with behavior problems is of major concern in the therapeutic process; that is, his environment is central to his immediate treatment as well as to his long-term adjustment. This fact, as suggested, constitutes a tenet of behavior modification. Generally, the most significant events in the patient's environment—events that can affect his behavior—are the activities of other people. Those with the greatest potential for influencing his behaviors are individuals with whom he has direct and very frequent contact; their activities contribute most to strengthening and weakening his various behaviors. Because the nurse is in the unique position of having the most significant number of contacts with the hospitalized individual, she/he can be the major treatment agent in the behavior modification program.[3] The behaviors of the nurse form a significant portion of the hospitalized patient's environment and, therefore, has primary importance in the remediation of his difficulties.

The activities of the nurse who deals with patients in the home environment and in other nonhospital settings or who deals with children in school situations also are related significantly to helping individuals with behavior problems. The contact that the nurse in a community setting has with a particular patient, however, is not likely to be as continuous as it is in a hospital or in another institution. For this reason, the nurse in the community or school situation can enhance her effectiveness by teaching those in continuous contact with the patient to become *part of* the treatment program. Most nurses can enlist the help of resource personnel, such as family members or foster grandparents; they can become involved in giving

---

[3]The author recognizes that there are many excellent male as well as female nurses; but since the majority of nurses are women, he will use hereafter the feminine pronouns, "she and her," in this book to refer to all nurses. This practice is merely for the sake of convenience and should not be taken as an indication of sexism in any form on the author's part.

health care services. This curative and preventative step along with a demonstration of the utility of behavior modification procedures in health teaching will be discussed in Chapter 3.

It is often difficult to separate the teaching and treating activities of the nurse using behavior modification. To a large degree, she instructs the patient how to improve. Meaningful behavior modification, which results in durable and extensive changes, may involve teaching the patient to treat himself as well as teaching others to care for him.

The nurse can be involved in behavior modification programs for helping many individuals with differing behavior problems. The examples included in this book will suggest only a portion for which she will find behavior modification principles useful and the various settings in which she can carry out behavior modification programs. As will be shown, the nurse can incorporate behavioral principles for dealing with hospitalized patients and for treating individuals residing in the natural environment.

There are various functions the nurse can have in a behavior modification program. For instance, she may be in charge of designing and implementing a behavior modification program for a patient (e.g., see Aiken, 1970, Chapter 3, Section 3.6); she may be responsible for carrying out an already designed one supervised by a psychologist, psychiatrist, or social worker (see Applications 13 and 14); or she may be in charge of supervising one that another "helping agent" is putting into effect (see Chapter 3 Section 3.6).

In their description of a behavior modification ward for mental patients, Schaefer and Martin (1969), show that the staff nurse often needs to make quick decisions about such matters as when to provide a favorable consequence for an adaptive behavior. Therefore, the instructions that she receives from the psychiatrist should not be so specific that they curtail her freedom to make quick decisions or to be creative in formulating plans for changing activities. On the behavior modification unit that Schaefer and Martin described, nurses received only general directives concerning the overall behavior goals for the patient. From these instructions, nurses were expected to institute specific behavior modification programs.

To effectively utilize behavioral principles, the nurses on this ward had to coordinate their activities. For example, according to another report (Schaefer and Martin, 1966), nurses were able to observe and record the behaviors of 10 patients daily (Monday–Friday), 30 times each day. That is, they observed the behaviors of 10 patients once each half hour during all of the morning and most of the afternoon shifts, five days a week. The resultant observations were relatively detailed and complete. (Making behavioral observations is a necessary step in behavior modification.) After the nurses had gathered their notes, they and other staff members, who were in virtually continuous contact with the patients, effectively could modify "apathy" among the patients—20 were helped to become less apathetic as a result of behavior modification (see Chapter 6, Section 6.1).

In another example of a team effort, Fordyce et al. (1968) reported that chronic pain behaviors displayed by patients in a rehabilitation hospital could be treated by a team composed of physiatrists, occupational therapists, social workers, nurses, and others. Attending physicians monitored the behavior modification programs for every patient.

Turner (1970) has discussed a very exciting team approach to helping emotionally disturbed children. Members most frequently in contact with the children are nurses and child-care workers. Consequently, these professionals design, implement, and evaluate behavioral programs for the children under the guidance of a psychologist, who is the program director. According to Turner, other specialists (e.g., psychiatrists and special education teachers) provide valuable assistance in the behavioral treatment programs for each child; also, Turner notes that the parents of each child are taught to carry out behavior modification procedures. Teaching parents behavior modification is an extremely valuable tactic which can have long term benefits. In addition to applying behavior modification procedures, the nurses also promote physical health care measures for the children. This team approach, characterized by open lines of communication and by a direct interchange of ideas among the members, resembles the type of team that a good home provides for a child—the members providing treatment serve momentarily as parents for the child (Browning and Stover, 1971).

In sum, there are several ways a nurse can function in behavior modification when it is employed to help patients with varied behavior difficulties. As new models of nursing are advanced, especially those advocating increased autonomy, the possible ways nurses can use as well as function in behavior modification will increase.

The effective utilization of behavior modification as a tool for remediating behavior problems requires that the nurse maintain a high degree of accuracy, precision, methodicalness, flexibility, and creativity when she is designing, is implementing, and is evaluating behavior modification programs and when she is teaching others about behavior modification per se. Each patient needs to be considered separately in terms of *his* behavior problems and *his* responsiveness to the procedures useful in ameliorating behavior problems. One of the most important and frequently used procedures in a behavior modification program, for instance, is Positive Reinforcement, but different positive reinforcers may be necessary for different patients. What is a reinforcer for one patient and, therefore, effective in strengthening his behavior may not be a reinforcer for another patient and, therefore, is ineffective for him. If a behavior modification program is not fitted to the particular problems and preferences of the individual patient, it probably will be unsuccessful. Effective utilization of behavior modification also requires that the behavior modifier performs certain activities. The nurse herself can execute them as a member of a team or can supervise others in carrying them out; when the nurse teaches others behavior modification, these activities form the structure of what she teaches. They constitute the behavior modification process, outlined in the next section.

TERMS AND QUESTIONS

Terms

Behavior Problem

Questions

1. What is the behavioral position regarding the following statements, which refer to people with behavior problems?
   (a) Symptoms (behaviors) should not be the focus of treatment. One should treat the underlying disturbance that causes the symptoms.
   (b) "Symptom substitution" will be likely only if the symptoms are the major objectives in treatment.
   (c) Diagnosis as it is traditionally carried out for mentally ill people is a useful process.
2. What two explanations may a behaviorist give for the occurrence of what appears to be symptom substitution?
3. Generally, what information do behaviorists seek regarding an individual's problems?
4. In what ways can a nurse who uses behavior modification principles function in a behavior modification program?

1.2 *BEHAVIOR MODIFICATION*

A General Overview of the Behavior Modification Process

Behavior modification is a process for dealing with the socially relevant problems of human beings. It consists of three related stages: assessment, intervention, and evaluation. *Assessment* pertains to defining, observing, and recording problematic behavior for the patient as well as the events affecting this behavior. *Intervention* involves the application of specific behavior modification procedures for improving the patient's behavior in order that he can function more capably. *Evaluation* includes (1) closely monitoring the patient's progress during intervention, so that the effects of the behavior modification procedures on the patient can be scrutinized continuously—this step makes it possible to determine whether he is improving; (2) ascertaining whether the observations made about the patient's behavior are accurate; (3) determining whether the behavior modification procedures have caused the positive changes in the patient's behavior; (4) finding out how long improvement lasts after treatment ends (*follow-up evaluation*).

Thus, a nurse should make certain that the patient's behaviors are accurately defined as well as precisely observed and recorded, and that the behavior modification program is skillfully designed and critically evaluated—evaluation includes continually monitoring the patient's progress in treatment. The nurse in the institutional setting can carry out these activities herself or can teach aides and other personnel to help. In the community or in the school, the nurse may want to focus on teaching the patient, his family members, or other individuals involved with him about behavior modification treatment practices; *or she may use behavior modification principles for health teaching.* She facilitates the treatment of any patient and enhances the likelihood of preventing future difficulties if she enlists the aid of individuals who are, or whom she can make, a significant part of the patient's daily environment.

Central to the nurse's activities in instituting the behavior modification process is her realization that the problems people have—whether labeled normal, neurotic, or psychotic—can all be translated into behaviors provided that these problems are carefully assessed. Rather than to ask what the patient is (e.g., Is he schizophrenic, Is he normal?), it is in the best interests of the patient to observe what he does (e.g., Does he interact with other people?). Understanding what a patient does and, inversely, what he doesn't do is vital.

Each of the stages of the behavior modification process will be detailed in this book, but the major emphasis will be on intervention. Thus, Chapters 3 and 4 will describe the procedures most useful to nurses, and Chapter 5 will present the techniques involved in assessment and in evaluation.

Judgments about Behavior and Behavior Modification

All forms of treatment for patients, at some point, involve judgments: what to treat, how to treat, when to treat, the effectiveness and meaningfulness of treatment, and so on. For example, judging effectiveness is related to how much change takes place in a patient's behavior (Baer, Wolf, and Risley, 1968). Alterations comprehensive enough so that he is helped to behave more capably determine whether a nurse can decide if behavior modification has been effective for the patient. Of course, to say that a patient is behaving more capably is a judgment that nurses and other individuals closely associated with the patient must make based on their knowledge of what capable behavior in a particular situation, such as functioning adequately in a mental hospital, really means (Baer, Wolf, and Risley, 1968). Similarly, the nurse has to judge whether the behavior modification program was meaningful. The requirements for this aspect will be discussed in Chapter 3.

As indicated in Section 1.1, socially relevant problems are those that most individuals, including the patient, consider as such. These judgments reflect the values of the judges. And the values in turn reflect the standards of the society in which the judges live. At different times in history or in various cultures during the same period of time, a specific behavior may be considered abnormal or normal and, thereby, in need of change or not in need of change. What was considered undesirable or deviant during one period (e.g., a butch haircut on a man in the eighteenth century) might be sanctioned and considered desirable at a later time in history (e.g., a butch haircut in the 1950's). Today, styles are different and deviancy is attributed to some behaviors desirable in the past and vice versa. Similarly, what is labeled abnormal in one society may not be labeled abnormal in another. Thus, for the Australian aborigine, undergoing or performing a subincision rite is normal behavior; but for the average American, this activity would be judged grossly deviant.

Therefore, the designation of behavior as problematic, abnormal, or undesirable and conversely, the designation of behavior as normal and desirable are social culturally based judgments—that is, they primarily result from the cultural standards with which we have been imbued. *Desirable* and *undesirable*, the terms used to describe behavior in this book, do not represent qualities differentiating behaviors from one another—the procedures effective in changing one are the same as the procedures effective in changing the other. Undesirable behavior is not different from desirable behavior except that society's members (e.g., the individual patient and the nurse) condemn one and approve of the other.

It should be reiterated that very often the individual patient (e.g., the mental or the retarded patient) and the treatment expert disagree about which behaviors should be approved of and which behaviors should be condemned. For example, the mental patient may attempt to kill himself, and the nurse will attempt to prevent him. To treat a patient for behavior problems he wants left alone is a knotty problem that often, justly or unjustly, is resolved by declaring him currently incapable of making important decisions for himself. Thus, many mental and retarded patients are judged unable to determine for themselves what behaviors they should be taught or even what their problems are. The staff caring for these patients may choose to enhance their decision-making abilities—a staff decision predicated on the judgment that independent decision making is desirable.

Treatment Approaches for Reducing Fears and Anxieties

Behavior modification has developed from several sources. Particularly valuable have been the contributions of operant learning and respondent conditioning. This book will deal mainly with the operant learning principles and behaviors called *operants*. These are the behaviors of most concern to nurses who care for individuals with behavior problems. *Respondent* behaviors and the procedures applicable to modifying them, however, are also important to nurses and, therefore, will be covered briefly in this chapter.

Several differences exist between these two classes of behavior. First, speaking informally, *respondents are involuntary activities whereas operants are usually voluntary ones.* For example, salivating with food in your mouth is a respondent; you can't stop yourself from salivating under this condition by simply telling yourself that you are not going to salivate. Your salivation is involuntary. Reaching for gauze is an operant. Holding out your hand appears to be a voluntary activity. Operants, however, are not capricious behaviors. Once the events affecting them are delineated, they are as predictable and as controllable as respondents. Second, *respondents are elicited by events (stimuli) that precede them.* When food, a stimulus, is placed in your mouth, you salivate. Operants are not elicited. Just how operants can be made to occur and can be weakened or strengthened will be discussed in Chapters 3 and 4. Third, *respondents, in contrast to operants, are usually unaffected by events (stimuli) that follow them—the events that occur after a respondent usually do not affect it.* Thus, if someone strikes your knee (patellar tendon) with a hammer, your leg will jerk. The leg-jerk is a respondent caused by someone striking your knee. Whether or not a $10 prize is given to those who exhibit the leg-jerk in response to the knee-tap will not alter the likelihood that the leg-jerk respondent will occur when the knee is tapped. Operants, on the other hand, are strongly affected by events that follow them—a $10 prize for the performance of some operant would be likely to increase the strength of that behavior.

Human behavior is very complex, and any sequence of activities, such as a child's touching a hot stove, his crying, and his running first to his mother and then to his father, involves both operants and respondents. Nevertheless, the procedures of behavior modification based on operant learning can be applied to improving most human behavior.

Before we discuss these procedures, we shall consider treatment approaches that can be used to modify respondent behaviors, namely anxiety and fear, that are labeled as emotional. To understand how these behaviors can arise, we will briefly examine *respondent conditioning.*

Respondent conditioning, at times, called Pavlovian or classical conditioning, was systematically investigated during the early part of this century by a Russian physiologist named Ivan Petrovich Pavlov. Basically, respondent conditioning involves the attachment of respondent behaviors to certain stimuli. The stimuli to which respondents are attached—the stimuli that can be made to elicit the desired behavior—are originally unable to elicit it. Ringing a bell initially will not cause a dog to salivate. But food in his mouth will.

Through respondent conditioning, however, neutral stimuli, such as a bell, can come to elicit respondents, such as salivation.

To understand this process, consider the following facts:

(1) Some stimuli can elicit certain involuntary reactions without any conditioning being necessary. The relationship between a particular stimulus and an activity is inborn. For example, food in the mouth causes salivation; dust in your eye will cause tears to flow; a blow to your patellar tendon with a hammer will cause your leg to jerk; a light shining on the pupil of your eye will cause your pupil to contract; a loud noise can cause blood vessels to constrict; certain stimuli can cause blood vessels to dilate resulting in a person becoming flushed. These stimuli, which from birth automatically cause certain respondents to occur, are called *unconditional stimuli.*

(2) *A neutral stimulus* and an unconditional stimulus may be presented at almost the same time, and the involuntary reaction automatically elicited by the unconditional stimulus alone will still occur. Thus, ringing a bell and food in the mouth, two stimuli, can be presented at the same time and salivation will still occur. (The ringing bell will not cause salivation before conditioning and hence is called a neutral stimulus.) *If a neutral stimulus is presented just before the unconditional stimulus—and both these stimuli are presented in this manner enough times—eventually the neutral stimulus alone will be able to elicit the involuntary behavior.* Thus, if a bell is rung just before food is placed in a dog's mouth, then, after a number of these stimulus pairings, the ringing bell alone will elicit salivation. This procedure is respondent conditioning. The previously neutral stimulus, which can now elicit the involuntary activity is called a *conditional stimulus.* (The terms *conditioned* and *unconditioned* are found in most books and articles concerned with respondent conditioning; these terms are used in the same way as *conditional* and *unconditional.* An error in translation from Russian to English is responsible for the popularity of conditioned and unconditioned as opposed to the more accurate words conditional and unconditional.)

There are some respondents, such as fear and anxiety, that can be elicited by presenting conditional stimuli. (In the following discussion, no distinction will be made between these two reactions.) An individual is not born fearful of the sights and smells in a physician's office. This reaction, however, can become attached to the smells and the appearance of a physician's office through respondent conditioning. Painful stimuli, unconditional stimuli (e.g., receiving an injection) can elicit fear. If the painful stimulus and the smell in a physician's office occur together enough times, then the smell by itself can elicit fear. Thus, it can be attached to stimuli that are not its inborn sources. Watson and Raynor (1920), in a classic study, demonstrated experimentally that a small child could come to fear furry objects, such as a rat or rabbit, that originally did not elicit fear. By allowing a child to play with a furry animal and then by making a loud noise, the authors could induce their subject to fear furry animals. The loud noise was an unconditional stimulus for fear.

The main point is that a wide variety of situations can cause fear or anxiety and, thereby, induce what is frequently called an emotional state. Medical equipment in a hospital or the thought of being in an elevator or being touched by another person can cause fear or anxiety for some people; the respondent conditioning process is involved in this learning.

There are various behavior modification approaches for helping individuals who experience fear and anxiety when confronted with stimuli, such as heights, wide spaces, needles, medical equipment in a hospital, the thought of being in a hospital, and other stimuli. Several of these behavior modification approaches attempt to break the link between the specific stimuli (e.g., doctor's office) and the emotional respondents (e.g., fear) by connecting new reactions that are incompatible with the emotional respondents. Thus, if the thought of simply being inside a hospital elicits intense fear, an attempt is made to condition relaxation responses to this thought. Relaxation and fear are incompatible; they cannot both occur at the same time. If relaxation can gradually be strengthened, and fear can gradually be weakened, the thought of being inside a hospital and even walking inside one will no longer elicit fear. (There are various responses incompatible with fear, such as eating and relaxing.)

Jones (1924) was able to reduce fear in a child by feeding him in the presence of the object he feared. It was brought into the room where the child was eating and was placed far away from him. Slowly the object was moved closer and closer to the child while he was eating. Gradually, the fear attached to the object was reduced. Conquering fears in this way involves some important elements. First, a response incompatible with fear or anxiety must be selected. Relaxation and the pleasant responses accompanying eating may be used. Second, the feared object must be gradually introduced. Thus, if a person is afraid of dogs, a dog should not be suddenly dropped into his lap. It should be introduced step by step. Perhaps a small dog can be brought into the room and placed 20 feet away from the person. Then the dog can be brought progressively closer to the individual, until he encounters little or no fear. Other strategies are possible, but the gradual introduction of the feared object is essential while the individual is either relaxed, is eating or is engaged in some other pleasant activity.

One of the most frequently used behavior therapy techniques, which incorporates these elements, is known as *systematic desensitization.* It was developed by Dr. Joseph Wolpe, a psychiatrist. According to Wolpe and Lazarus (1966), if incompatible responses that inhibit anxiety can be made to occur in the presence of the stimuli that elicit the anxiety, the bond between these stimuli and the anxiety will be weakened. With this technique, each patient is taught how to relax the various parts of his body. In addition, the stimulus eliciting anxiety is broken down into elements and is arranged in an ascending order from least to most anxiety producing. Thus, if an individual fears wide open spaces, the elements of this reaction—from stepping outside the front door, for example, to walking down a wide street—are ordered in a hierarchy based on interviews and various other assessment devices. Each component of the fear, that is, each situation causing it, is arranged in order of the amount it elicits. Finally, the patient is told to relax and to imagine one of the scenes from the hierarchy. *Beginning with the least* anxiety producing and *ending with the most* anxiety producing, the scenes are presented to the patient. Advancing from one scene to the next on the hierarchy is done only when the fear associated with the previous scene has dissipated. Thus, anxiety is always kept at a minimum, whereas relaxation is kept at a maximum. By slowly moving up the hierarchy and by backtracking when the individual reports too much anxiety, the therapist is able to help the patient conquer his fears.

Nurses may use procedures based on the ones just outlined. For example, Aiken (1970) has suggested that pre-operative teaching may involve a form of desensitization entailing a graded exposure to increasingly threatening events. Thus, a patient may first be taken to an empty recovery room containing various medical equipment. Next, the patient may return to the recovery room during the time when some moderately ill people are there. After this step, the nurse may accompany the patient back to the recovery room in the height of the busy period, when he can see some seriously ill people. Presumably, the patient's conversations with the nurse will be pleasurable during each of these encounters and will be incompatible with the fear these situations elicit. The pleasant responses, therefore, may be made to predominate over the anxiety reactions. During this procedure, if the patient becomes too anxious, verbal hierarchies should be arranged before the nurse actually takes the patient to the recovery room (Aiken, 1970). Furthermore, Aiken wisely cautions that the anxiety hierarchies, which are constructed, should be based on the specific details of what the patient fears and not on what the nurse believes that he probably fears. Techniques that incorporate a gradual exposure to increasingly fear-producing situations can be employed also in the mental hospital (e.g., Schaefer and Martin, 1969).

Thus, there are approaches for reducing fears and anxieties elicited by various stimuli. The procedures applicable to changing these respondent behaviors, however, will not be discussed further in this book. For the nurse interested in pursuing this area, selections are listed in the supplementary reading section for Chapter 1. The nurse involved in ongoing patient care is likely to find that in her interactions with patients the procedures pertinent to modifying operant behaviors are useful more frequently than methods relating to altering respondent reactions.

Some Additional Comments about Emotions

Emotions such as fear, anxiety, anger, aggression, sadness, love, and joy are very complex responses that have both internal components (e.g., changes in the size of blood-vessels) and external behavioral components (e.g., smiling, crying). Emotions are difficult to investigate because these components cannot always be accurately observed. For example, if an individual has tears in his eyes, you don't know for certain from this information alone whether he is sad or is overjoyed, whether he is crying for attention or whether he has just been peeling onions. Crying when you are happy differs from crying when you are sad. And both these tearful responses differ from the crying of a child who is neither happy nor in pain but who merely wants attention from his mother.

When we label a response emotional, we are not only looking at it, but we also are looking at the situation which caused it. Thus, if a loved one in a friend's family has died, we probably will say that our friend's tears reflect his sadness (emotion). But if we know that our friend has dust under his contact lens, we will not call his tears an emotional response. The *situation* eliciting the response, as well as the response, determine whether we use the word emotional or some name of an emotion (e.g., sadness) to describe an individual's behavior (Bijou and Baer, 1961).

Being able to say that a patient is angry or sad, however, is not nearly as useful for the nurse as being able to predict what the patient will do under a given set of circumstances. Knowing what the patient *is* (e.g., he is happy, he is sad) is not usually the most important information required to change his behavior. The most important information is obtained by assessing his activities and the conditions controlling them. For accuracy and precision, it is necessary to observe directly what he does, not to infer that he is angry or sad, and so forth.

Accurate assessment is the first step in improving the patient's behavior. Thus, rather than to say that he must be angry because he hits other patients, it is better to find out what situations may be causing or contributing to the hitting-behavior. Although rage may be present—it is difficult to know for certain—anger may not be causing the hitting any more than the hitting is causing the anger. Both the anger and the hitting are responses resulting from situations that the nurse eventually can understand by directly observing the patient's behavior in different circumstances.

Some Comments concerning Mental Hospitals

Because many examples of behavior modification, which will be presented in this book, concern patients in mental hospitals and in other institutions, we will examine briefly some of the problems inherent in institutions, particularly in mental hospitals. Behavior modification principles have been used in dealing with a number of the difficulties.

Books and articles have been written about the development of mental hospitals. Before Pinel and Dix, mental hospitals largely were pits wherein patients were brutally treated. The changeover from the inhumane handling of the mentally ill to current practices has been an improvement, of course, but the large mental hospitals of today still can have grievous effects on patients. Goffman (1961), in particular, has commented on the role of patients in modern mental hospitals and has painted rather an ugly picture of the *behavior deterioration* (loss of essential behaviors required for living in society) and the *disculturation* (loss of contact with the outside community, the family, and friends) that can take place. Goffman and other writers have discussed how the hospital routine often fosters conformity and passivity among patients and how the day-to-day problems of ward management often preempt treatment.

A patient who spends years in a mental hospital may be unable to leave it because he has lost many of the behaviors necessary for functioning adequately in the outside community. In fact, he can become so removed from society that he can't re-enter even though his original behavior problems, that is, the activities resulting in his being hospitalized, are no longer present. Often, as the years the patient spends inside the mental hospital increase, the attention from his family and his friends decreases, and the constructive behaviors he once may have possessed evidence a progressive decay (Ayllon and Azrin, 1968).

Behavior modification principles have been applied in mental hospitals and have been directed at these problems. Major goals of programs have been to foster adaptive activities, to prevent behavior deterioration, and to help a patient re-enter the outside community. By helping him to reduce his behavior problems and to continue functioning in an adaptive manner while he is in the hospital and by discharging him when his problems have diminished sufficiently, the hospital staff can be instrumental in preventing behavior deterioration and disculturation (Ayllon and Azrin, 1968). The usefulness of *token reinforcement programs* in the application of behavior modification principles to institutionalized patients will be discussed in Chapter 7. These programs create environments that are responsive to a patient's desirable behaviors.

TERMS AND QUESTIONS

Terms

Behavior deterioration
Disculturation
Assessment
Intervention
Evaluation
Follow-up evaluation
Desirable behavior
Undesirable behavior
Operants
Respondents
Respondent conditioning
Unconditional stimulus
Neutral stimulus
Conditional stimulus
Systematic desensitization

Questions

1. What part do value judgments play in the designation of behavior as desirable or undesirable?
2. How may you reduce a patient's fear of needles?
3. What are some of the major differences between the operant of studying for an exam, and the respondent of experiencing anxiety at the thought of taking an exam?
4. Toward what goal have behavior modification programs in mental hospitals been directed?

1.3 *A SYNTHESIS*

Chapter 1 has had several objectives. One was to contrast the behavioral and the traditional approaches to those many human difficulties termed behavior problems. It has been argued that behavior problems should be treated directly and should not be by-passed in an effort to treat any hypothesized inner determinant of them. Symptom substitution, if any, was considered more the result of inadequate and incomplete treatment or of encountering new stresses than a phenomenon related to overlooking underlying causes.

Diagnosing behavior problems in the sense of categorizing someone as belonging to a certain class (e.g., schizophrenic) was rejected in favor of assessing his behavior and the events affecting it. There are negative effects associated with labeling a patient. And since these diagnostic designations, in addition, may be inaccurate, it seems wise to dispense with them.

It also was pointed out that behaviors considered desirable or undesirable are judged by individuals who reflect the values of their culture. No difference in kind exists between desirable and undesirable behavior but only between behavior approved of and behavior condemned by society during a given period. This truth implies that the basic procedures effective in altering any behavior will be effective in modifying undesirable behavior.

Another objective of this chapter was to outline some situations in which nurses can employ behavior modification principles and a number of the ways in which nurses can function in behavior modification. It was pointed out that when a nurse is either implementing or is supervising the implementation of a behavior modification program, she must make certain of the following: that the patient's behavior is defined, observed, and recorded accurately and precisely and that his behavior modification program is designed skillfully and is evaluated critically. Ably designing a behavior modification program for a patient requires that he be viewed as an individual who may have preferences and needs different from those of other patients. The procedures of behavior modification are applicable to most patients, but the specific variables (e.g., reinforcers) crucial for successful implementation often need to be tailored to the individual.

A major component of the nurse's activities in behavior modification is her ability to translate the patient's problems into observable behaviors. Making untestable inferences about "what patients are" (e.g., the patient is schizophrenic) are not as useful as finding out about "what patients do" (e.g., the patient shouts obscenities 30 times a day).

A further objective of this chapter was to define behavior modification as a three-staged process (assessment, intervention, evaluation) applicable in dealing with the socially relevant problems of human beings. In addition, it was pointed out that behavior cannot be thoroughly understood independent from either environmental events that precede it or from ones that follow it. As stated, a relationship exists between changes in the environment and changes in behavior. The behavior modification procedures discussed in the ensuing chapters of this book capitalize on this fact of life and, thereby, may be used to help individuals behave more capably than before.

The final objective of this chapter was to mention the differences between respondent and operant behaviors and to discuss treatment approaches useful in reducing respondents—for example, anxiety and fear—that are called emotions. It was indicated that respondents are involuntary behaviors caused by stimuli preceding them; operants, on the other hand, can be described as voluntary behaviors controlled, to a large extent, by their consequences. The effects of environment on operant behaviors will be discussed fully in Chapter 3.

Respondent conditioning was briefly outlined as a process explaining how respondents, such as fear and anxiety, become attached to stimuli, such as needles or heights, which are not inborn elicitors of fear. Ways of eliminating fears and anxieties as responses to conditional stimuli also were outlined. These approaches involve the connection of new reactions, such as relaxation, to the fear-producing stimuli; the new responses are incompatible with fear. When the patient imagines components of the feared situation or when he actually participates in it, he can experience a reduction in fear—provided that the situation is introduced gradually, in small portions, during times when he is relaxed or is experiencing pleasure of some sort. The potential value of this approach in pre-operative teaching has been suggested.

It was indicated, however, that procedures attempting to change operant behaviors are more pertinent to the activities of the nurse-practitioner. These techniques will be emphasized throughout this book.

Other topics were considered in this chapter: the impact of the mental hospital on the activities of the patient; the utility of directly assessing the patient's observable behaviors as well as the situations that affect them, rather than determining if certain emotions, believed to be reflected by his behaviors, are present.

In short, Chapter 1 has introduced some important issues and topics—several of which will be discussed more thoroughly later. In the next chapter, other issues relevant to behavior modification will be briefly examined.

SUPPLEMENTARY READINGS

CAHOON, D. D. "Symptom Substitution and the Behavior Therapies," *Psychological Bulletin*, 69, 1968, 149–156.

LAZARUS, A. A. "The Treatment of a Sexually Inadequate Man," in *Case Studies in Behavior Modification*, eds. L. P. Ullmann and L. Krasner. New York: Holt, Rinehart & Winston, Inc., 1965.

NEURINGER, C. "Behavior Modification as the Clinical Psychologist Views it," in *Behavior Modification in Clinical Psychology*, eds. C. Neuringer and J. Michael. New York: Appleton-Century-Crofts, 1970.

RACHMAN, S. "Systematic Desensitization," *Psychological Bulletin*, 67, 1967, 93–103.

STUART, R. B. *Trick or Treatment: How and When Psychotherapy Fails.* Champaign, Illinois: Research Press, 1970, pp. 5–120.

ULLMANN, L. P. AND L. KRASNER, eds. *Case Studies in Behavior Modification.* New York: Holt, Rinehart & Winston, Inc., 1965, pp. 1–29.

two Some Other Issues concerning Behavior Modification

2.1 *FORMULATING THE OBJECTIVES OF A BEHAVIOR MODIFICATION PROGRAM, THE WELFARE OF THE PATIENT, THE HUMAN RELATIONSHIP, EVALUATION AND MOTIVATION*

Some of the issues discussed in this brief chapter, which are similar to those examined in Chapter 1, (e.g., diagnosis), concern matters involving the duties and the obligations of the nurse in relation to the patient. Other issues (e.g., motivation) are mentioned primarily to alter misconceptions and to clarify the behavior modification point of view.

Stating the Goals for a Behavior Modification Program

The goals for a behavior modification program are the particular changes in the patient's activities that the nurse attempts to bring about through intervention. As will be indicated in Chapters 3 and 5, the objectives must be stated clearly before any attempt is made to change the patient's behavior.

In fact, the goals for a behavior modification program, once formulated, usually suggest the procedures that should be implemented. Thus, if an aim were to increase self-esteem, the procedures that should be used would be different from those employed if the objective were to decrease shouting obscenities; to increase the strength of one particular behavior entails steps different from those used to decrease the strength of another behavior.

The goals of a behavior modification program, once formulated, are not immutable. If at a later date acquired information reveals that the goals for a patient are inadequate or that other ones would be more suitable, changes should be made. Altering goals will be minimized, however, if the nurse carefully assesses the patient's problems before intervention is attempted.

Nor are behavior modification procedures immutable once they are implemented. If by monitoring the patient's behaviors during intervention, the nurse discovers that the procedures are not working correctly, she must make changes in them. This flexibility is an important feature of behavior modification. Continuous observation of the patient's behaviors provides the nurse with feedback concerning her methods and, thereby, allows her to institute beneficial alterations in the program as they become necessary.

Two important questions associated with setting goals for a patient are: What should the goals be? Who should help the patient achieve these goals? As stated previously, value judgments enter in when behavior is designated as desirable or undesirable and, therefore, become considerations when goals are formulated, because these goals are desirable changes in behavior. The aims of a behavior modification program must be beneficial to the patient in terms of his living more capably in society. But *who* can determine *what* living more capably in society really means for the individual? For example, consider the care of women who cannot adjust to the role of housewife. Should they be taught to adjust, or should they be taught how to help change society's view of the role of women? The individual with behavior problems, in the community, can decide which alterations in his behavior are necessary to increase his capabilities. And helping him to make informed choices is one obligation of the professional (Bandura, 1969).

The mental patient in a hospital or the retardate in an institution, on the other hand, often is unable to make informed choices about the necessary goals. For these individuals, the professional must, as a representative of society, make decisions about objectives (Ullmann and Krasner, 1965). When the patient is too "sick" or too retarded to decide what the objectives for his betterment should be, then the professionals responsible for his treatment become the primary decision makers; they must formulate the goals necessary for helping the patient lead a "better" existence than before.

If behavior changes are made without the permission of the patient, the professionals who define the goals must be explicit about what they intend to do so that *inspection by others* becomes possible. When the aims are made open to examination and to review, the danger of misusing behavior modification or any other procedure for selfish ends is reduced (Ball, 1968). The goals, as indicated, must be specified for technical reasons as well. We must be clear and definitive about what we intend to do for the individual.

The question of who should help the patient to achieve the goals in behavior modification has become a question that should be rephrased: Who is likely to be successful in helping the patient achieve the goals of a behavior modification program? In principal, the people most closely involved with the patient's daily activities are in the best position to help him. Therefore, several helping agents (e.g., the family) may be incorporated into a total treatment program for the patient. As suggested in Chapter 1, as the direct and continuous contact of the nurse with the patient becomes lessened, the utilization of other helping agents becomes increasingly necessary for effective treatment, for dealing with relapses after treatment, and for preventing the occurrence of new problems.

The Welfare of the Patient and Behavior Modification

Treatment professionals agree that the welfare of the patient is of primary concern. The differences among the various professionals are related mostly to their methods for helping the patient. The behavior modification method has often been criticized for not being geared toward the patient's welfare. Four issues related to this criticism will be dealt with here.

DEPRIVATION. *Deprivation* is a term in behavior modification that describes a process for increasing the effectiveness of a reward (reinforcer) at a particular time. (*Positive reinforcer* and *reward* are terms that often can be used interchangeably. But reward is more informal and less technically precise than reinforcer; also, reinforcer is more likely to be found in textbooks and in journals that deal with behavior modification. Consequently, in the ensuing pages of this text, reinforcer will gradually supplant reward.) Deprivation can be illustrated by the following example: Food is a reinforcer that an individual will attempt to obtain if he is hungry. Thus, if you have not eaten for awhile—if you have been temporarily deprived of food—you will take the time to prepare a meal for yourself (behaviors) and to set the dinner table (other behaviors). In short, you will engage in behaviors that result in obtaining the reinforcer, food; the effectiveness of food as a reinforcer for these behaviors is related to how hungry you are. On the other hand, if you have just eaten—you are no longer food deprived—food temporarily will lose its rewarding effect; under these conditions, you are likely not to engage in behaviors such as cooking and setting the table because you are no longer hungry. Being hungry and being food deprived are statements that mean the same.[1] Food becomes a more effective reinforcer for engaging in certain behaviors, if you are hungry (food deprived).

Reinforcers are important in helping patients to change their behavior. The deprivation process and the necessity of employing reinforcers for modifying behavior is discussed fully in Chapter 3. In addition, the utility of reinforcement in improving patients' behavior is documented throughout this book. The point to be made here, however, is the following: *Because administering reinforcers is so important in helping individuals to behave more capably, a process that makes these reinforcers effective, namely, deprivation, is vital.*

The ethical justification for initially depriving patients of some rewarding objects or activities so that you can give it to them later following desirable behavior, lies in the worthiness of this outcome in relation to the undesirability of deprivation considered by itself. As Cahoon (1968) has stated:

> . . . The ethical justification for any technique must lie in the value of the outcome relative to the severity or undesirability of the procedure considered by itself. Amputation to "cure" a hangnail would be unethical, but amputation would scarcely be unethical if necessary to arrest a gangrenous process.[2]

---

[1]But note that *food deprivation* is preferable to the term *hunger* because the former precisely specifies an environmental event which makes food an effective reinforcer.

[2]Delwin D. Cahoon, "Issues and implications of operant conditioning: Balancing procedures against outcomes," *Hospital and Community Psychiatry*, 19, 1968, 228.

Thus, the welfare of the patient may depend on a somewhat onerous procedure such as deprivation. In actuality, deprivation in the mental hospitals or in the institutions for the retarded may be equated with the controlled administration of reinforcers (Ball, 1968) and not with the denial of food, of medical treatment, or of adequate living quarters. Extrinsic rewards, such as food, eventually become unnecessary as the patient improves. Also, as will be shown later, deprivation of a rewarding activity, such as going to a movie, can simply mean that you limit the patient's access to this activity only for a very short time until he progresses in some small way. In fact, it can be stated as a general rule that if deprivation becomes extreme without the patient responding appropriately, then something is wrong with the behavior modification procedure being tried.

From the above, it is evident that judiciously using deprivation, as applied in behavior modification, is humane. Failing to control reinforcers, in contrast, may be harmful to a patient's welfare. It is definitely more compassionate to help a patient by implementing techniques that function to improve his condition than by not using them, thereby leaving the patient unchanged. Not extracting a diseased tooth because you believe it unmerciful to cause an individual discomfort would be a very inhumane belief with disastrous consequences for many people. Thus, if a procedure appears undesirable, it must be evaluated in terms of the good it can do for a patient relative to its own undesirability as a procedure, along with the possibility of employing alternative procedures that yield positive effects.

Rewarding Behavior Is Not Bribery. This issue concerns the use of extrinsic rewards such as money and food for individuals, especially for children. Parents and teachers often refer to this kind of reward, employed to develop desirable behaviors, as bribery. To call this bribery, however, is not only a denial of what generally takes place in society but is also an incorrect conceptualization of behavior modification practices.

Teachers, parents, employers, to name only a few, often give rewards. Teachers grade their students; parents buy toys for their children; and employers pay their employees. Often, however, these rewards do not systematically or do not consistently follow desirable behavior. This fact is unfortunate because rewarding behavior systematically and consistently, which will be discussed in Chapter 3, is the most efficient way to strengthen desirable behavior. When people object to the behavior modification practice of rewarding behavior by calling it bribery, they really must be objecting to systematically and consistently rewarding behavior, because everyone gives and receives rewards though, at times, this practice is done inefficiently. If the systematic and consistent administration of rewards for all behaviors suddenly ended, many individuals would be angry. If your employer, for instance, told you to come to work and that sometimes you would be paid and sometimes you wouldn't or that you would no longer be paid at all, you would probably quit. Similarly, it is doubtful whether an individual who has provided you with a service, such as painting your house, would be grateful if you told him that you might pay him in three years. Thus, to be consistent and systematic in rewarding behavior is simply to be efficient in encouraging and in developing behavior. Parents and teachers can do much for their children along these lines.

Perhaps, the major reason for discounting the appellation of bribery is that it really means something else. According to Webster, a bribe is "money or favor bestowed on or promised to a person in a position of trust *to pervert his judgment or corrupt his conduct.*"

Behavior modification, as a helping tool, does not pervert judgment or corrupt conduct but, rather, strengthens desirable conduct and weakens undesirable conduct. If external incentives (e.g., food, toys, or money) can operate in this fashion, they should be employed. A goal of behavior modification, however, is to help an individual become independent of these somewhat artificial reinforcers by bringing him into touch with different kinds (more natural) reinforcers, such as the praise and attention of other people, the feeling of accomplishment, or the enjoyment of the desirable behavior itself. These kinds of reinforcers are crucial to long-term improvement. As will be shown, the use of simpler rewards (e.g., food, toys, or money) may be the initial step, though temporary, in helping the patient come into touch with more naturally occurring reinforcers —that is, with reinforcers commonly used in our society.

THE ISSUE OF CONTROLLING THE PATIENT'S BEHAVIOR. Few nurses would disagree with the statement that the activities of the nurse influence those of the patient. The behavior modification position is that helping the patient to change in desirable ways involves altering his environment to influence his conduct beneficially. Behaviorists also maintain that it is wise to be explicit about what you do for the patient when you attempt to influence him; that is, it is not in the best interests of the patient to rely on procedures you have difficulty explaining precisely or managing effectively. Although the word *influence* is more benign than the word *control,* it also is less explicit. Consequently, behavior modifiers frequently use the latter term (control) when describing the effects of the environment, or more specifically, the results of planned changes in the environment (among which are the reactions of the behavior modifier) on the patient's behavior. (Both terms, however, are used in this book.)

The word *control* is objectionable to many people because it has been associated with brainwashing and with the punitive techniques of despots. But to say that all control is bad is to deny the positive effects of treatment.

All techniques to some extent exert control, although they often differ. To do nothing beneficial for a patient but instead to allow him to deteriorate determines what eventually happens to him as much as do the effective efforts made to help him. To say that we don't control in any way is false. And to say that control over behavior is bad is too general and too incomplete to be accurate.

By carefully managing and by thoroughly understanding what she does, the nurse can help a patient to behave in desirable ways. A nurse's behavior (e.g., implementing treatment procedures) can exert control over a patient's behavior resulting in favorable or unfavorable consequences for the patient. In fact, it can be stated safely that the failure of a patient to acquire desirable behavior or to decrease performing undesirable behavior reflects an inadequate utilization of procedures as much as or more than anything exclusively attributable to him.

A complete understanding of the ways people can either purposefully or unintentionally control the behavior of others will lessen the likelihood of inappropriately using powerful regulating procedures. Control can be usefully exercised by a nurse who fully assesses a patient's behavior and who carefully considers the ways to improve it.

Control over behavior, however, is not a one-way street. The patient also controls the nurse's behavior. To effectively help the patient, as discussed previously, the nurse must be sensitive to his needs and preferences (Schaefer and Martin, 1969). When it is recognized that the patient and the nurse control each other, a more complete understanding of the term *control* becomes possible.

Of all the procedures that can be used to control a patient's behavior, those based on rewards are the most powerful. The punitive techniques so often associated with control do not have the enduring influence or the beneficial possibilities of the rewarding ones. (Schaefer and Martin, 1969). *Positive Reinforcement,* based on the judicious application of reinforcers following behavior, will be stressed in this book.

In sum, control over behavior is associated with all treatment approaches and should not be construed automatically as undesirable. Furthermore, control definitely does not have one side—the nurse and the patient influence each other. Behavior modification is not brainwashing but is an approach that endeavors to help its recipients.

THE ISSUE CONCERNING THE HUMANENESS OF BEHAVIOR MODIFICATION. Behavior modification is an approach that can work quickly, effectively, and meaningfully; that can eventually furnish a patient with a sense of mastery over his problems; and that has the potential for providing a patient with the dignity of being able to treat himself (see concluding section). As Bandura (1969) points out, behavior modification may be used to remove restrictions limiting the personal freedom of the individual, such as deficiencies in behavior that preclude him from many opportunities, or excesses in deviant behavior that prohibit him from living competently. Behavior modification—indeed, a humane approach that can contribute significantly to the welfare of the patient—is direct and is supportive of his attempts to function more capably. The results of many examples included in this book and the effects of a multitude of other published reports not included herein support this assertion.

Evaluation in Behavior Modification

Evaluation, the third stage of behavior modification as outlined in Chapter 1, frequently is opposed on ethical grounds. Actually, there are four types of evaluation that can be carried out in behavior modification, and objections generally pertain to only one of these, namely, whether treatment procedures were responsible for changes in the patient's behavior. The other three evaluations involve: monitoring the behavior of the patient during the intervention stage so that ineffective procedures can be abandoned and effective ones can be implemented; determining if the observations that one nurse makes agree with the observations that a second nurse makes; finding out how long improvement lasts after treatment ends (i.e., follow-up). It is unlikely that objections concerning the value of monitoring the patient's progress will occur, because this assessment, quite obviously, relates to his welfare. Also, the other two steps are unlikely to be opposed seriously because accuracy and thoroughness, as most people would agree, are important in treatment. Although these last two stages are often omitted, their completion is not viewed as detrimental to the patient's welfare.

Many professionals, however, consider the remaining type of

evaluation antithetical to the patient's welfare, because evaluating whether the treatment procedures caused the changes in his behavior customarily has involved a temporary reinstatement of his problem. There exist, however, other approaches that do not involve this objectionable feature. These other methods evaluate *by adding to and by refining the positive effects of the procedures* (see Chapter 5, Section 5.4).

Evaluation of treatment procedures is an important step in behavior modification not only for the welfare of the individual being treated but also for the welfare of the many patients yet to be treated. Future use should be related to knowledge the nurse has acquired concerning the effectiveness of these methods with previous patients. Ignorance about the instrumental ways of caring for an individual with behavior problems can only impair his progress.

The Human Relationship

Behavior modification does not, as is commonly thought, dismiss the importance of the relationship a patient has with an individual helping him. Undoubtedly, the bond between a nurse and a patient can facilitate or can hinder the latter's progress with behavior modification procedures. And the relationship between a patient and a nurse can become more positive as the patient improves, that is, as the behavior modification procedures begin to have positive effects.

The nurse's behaviors essential in forming a good relationship with a patient are difficult to state definitively. It seems, however, that being systematic and consistent with the patient as well as demonstrating respect, civility and courtesy toward him (Gambrill, Thomas, and Carter, 1970) can influence the nurse-patient relationship and the success of the behavior modification program.

Motivation

Often patients in mental hospitals, especially, seem to be aimless and uninvolved in any activities. Many of the ones that nurses try to make palatable to patients (e.g., weekly dances, occupational therapy) are designed to reduce aimlessness. The involvement of patients in useful activities may be necessary for successful rehabilitation. But what facilitates any patient's involvement, and what causes his disinterest? The answers to these questions usually center around the term *motivation*.

Motivation is used to explain partially both patient activity and inactivity. Lack of motivation is reflected in his inactivity, and adequate motivation is reflected in his involvement. To rehabilitate a patient, it is necessary to motivate him (to remotivate him). According to Mereness and Karnosh (1966), remotivation "has as its purpose the stimulation of patients who have lost interest in reality and who have lost a sense of personal value."[3] Motivation, however, is not some internal energy that patients must possess in order to become better and is not some force that can be built up or can be diminished.

Motivation, related to behavior, in part refers to procedures that affect reinforcement; and reinforcement can markedly affect a patient's activity. More specifically, motivation deals with techniques that can make reinforcers more effective in strengthening behavior at a particular time (Reynolds, 1968). A strengthening of the important activities that constitute part of a rehabilitation program can occur if effective reinforcers are used systematically and consistently. Potent reinforcers can be employed to strengthen the behaviors that will help the patient regain both his "interest in reality" and his "sense of personal value."

We have already discussed one technique for making reinforcers more effective and, thereby, more instrumental in strengthening desirable behavior. This technique was called deprivation. By controlling the administration of reinforcers, the nurse can enhance their efficacy. In short, motivation is a term often applied when the effectiveness (potency) of reinforcers in strengthening desirable behavior is considered. How an event becomes a reinforcer in the first place can be explained by the principles of operant learning that form the bases of behavior modification (see Chapter 3). Motivation, as we have discussed it, simply describes technological details of how reinforcers can be made more effective (Reynolds, 1968).

The answer to the query about what a nurse can do to help a patient become more involved in the activities vital to his rehabilitation is the following: *develop a system providing a patient with incentives for engaging in adaptive behaviors.* If potent reinforcers are available, the behaviors will become strong and the likelihood of rehabilitation will increase. The durability of the adaptive activities; that is, the extent to which a patient demonstrates a persistency in engaging in them once they are strengthened (an indication of how "motivated" he is) is affected greatly by *how often* the potent

---

[3]Dorothy Mereness and Louis J. Karnosh, *Essentials of Psychiatric Nursing* (St. Louis, Missouri: The C. V. Mosby Company, 1966), p. 86.

reinforcers are provided; but the relationship between the frequency with which reinforcers are given and the persistence of behavior is not a simple one, as will be explained in Chapter 3, Section 3.5.

The task of rehabilitating patients in mental hospitals, in other institutions, or in the community is intertwined with developing a workable system of administering reinforcers for adaptive behaviors. Such a plan requires the use of potent reinforcers. As will be shown, there are numerous sources of reinforcement that can be brought to bear on the problems of all people. An environment that fosters adaptive behavior, a "motivating" environment, can be created on a large scale for mental patients and for other institutionalized individuals (see Chapter 7). This type of surrounding will capitalize on the varied, potent sources of reinforcement that can be tailored to fit the preferences of an individual patient and, thereby, can be instrumental in habilitating and rehabilitating persons with behavior problems.

TERMS AND QUESTIONS

Terms

Deprivation
Motivation

Questions

1. When must another individual (e.g., a nurse) set goals for the patient? What danger is there in this decision? How can the danger be minimized?
2. What do you think of the following statements?
   (a) Deprivation, in any form, is harmful to a patient and is an inhumane technique.
   (b) Rewarding behavior, in any form, is bribery.
3. Do all attempts to help a patient exert control over his behavior in some way, and is this control one sided (e.g., nurse over patient)?
4. What is the major value of being explicit about how we are going to help a patient?
5. Why is evaluating whether treatment procedures were responsible for changes in the patient's behavior important?
6. How can a patient's improvement affect his relationship with a nurse?

7. What is motivation? How may the nurse enhance the effectiveness of "rest" as a reinforcer?

2.2 *A SYNTHESIS*

Several issues were considered in this chapter. Motivation, for example, was discussed mainly with reference to increasing the potency of reinforcers.

In addition, it was shown that clear, explicit goals must be formulated for the patient in order that adequate behavior modification procedures, tailored to him, may be designed. Rigid adherence to goals or methods when evidence indicates the need for change was opposed. When the patient cannot formulate the appropriate goals for his own betterment, the treatment professional will have to assume this function, which makes the need for stating explicit goals even more important. After the objectives for helping the patient have been formulated, behavior modification procedures can be implemented.

The patient's welfare is of primary concern. Consequently, a thorough understanding of principles, such as deprivation and rewarding behavior, must be acquired in order not to dismiss them carelessly because, as processes, they are vital to patient care. Furthermore, it is important to recognize that controlling behavior is related to treating it and cannot be regarded as entirely negative. Regulating behavior is neither entirely "bad," nor one sided; the nurse and the patient affect each other's behavior. As stated, it is preferable to be explicit than to be vague about how we intend to control behavior; the danger of misusing powerful procedures that can check behavior becomes reduced if we are specific about them. By thoroughly understanding the patient's problems and the techniques she can apply to help him, the nurse can feel more confident that behavior modification will remain humane. It is an approach in which procedures for helping the patient can work quickly, effectively, and meaningfully; can furnish the patient with a sense of mastery over his problems; potentially, can provide the patient with the dignity of being able to care for himself. As with all other treatment and educational activities, however, it is possible to use behavior modification selfishly and foolishly.

Lack of information concerning the essentials of behavior modification will allow many to reject it as devoid of human relationships and of concern for the patient. To the elimination of this ignorance and its unfortunate consequence—the repudiation of a useful approach to helping people—our book is devoted.

Much of what has been said in this chapter (e.g., the need to evaluate behavior modification procedures and to employ potent reinforcers) will be repeated later. In the next chapter, the most important, flexible, and helpful procedure will be discussed, namely, Positive Reinforcement. As will be shown, Positive Reinforcement can be applied to remedy various behavior problems afflicting many individuals.

SUPPLEMENTARY READINGS

Bandura, A. *Principles of Behavior Modification.* New York: Holt, Rinehart & Winston, Inc., 1969, pp. 73–88.

O'Leary, K. D., R. Poulos, and V. T. Devine "Tangible Reinforcers: Bonuses or Bribes?" *Journal of Consulting and Clinical Psychology,* 38, 1972, 1–8.

Reynolds, G. S. *A Primer of Operant Conditioning.* Glenview, Illinois: Scott, Foresman and Company, 1968, pp. 118–130.

Risley, T. R. "Behavior Modification: An Experimental-Therapeutic Endeavor," in *Behavior Modification and Ideal Mental Health Services,* eds. L. A. Hamerlynck, P. O. Davidson, and L. E. Acker. Calgary, Alberta [Canada]: University of Calgary, 1969.

Skinner, B. F. "Freedom and the Control of Men," *American Scholar,* 25, 1955–1956, 47–65. (Also in B. F. Skinner, *Cumulative Record.* New York: Appleton-Century-Crofts, 1961.)

Ulrich, R., T. Stachnik, and J. Mabry, eds. *Control of Human Behavior: From Cure to Prevention,* Vol. 2. Glenview, Illinois: Scott, Foresman and Company, 1970, pp. 334–343, 347–358.

three | *Accelerating Desirable Behavior*

3.1 *FUNDAMENTAL TOPICS*

Behavior and Stimuli

As mentioned previously, a behavior is an activity that an individual performs. Swimming, eating, watching television, solving mathematical problems, using graphs for calculating the calorie intake of low-birth-weight babies, burglarizing houses, hallucinating, and shouting obscene language are all behaviors. Some are desirable, and some are not.

Some behaviors appear to be simple, such as putting a spoonful of food into your mouth, whereas others seem to be complex, such as caring for a child with a tracheo-esophageal fistula; the complexity of any activity relates to the abilities of the individual performing it. For example, self-feeding is difficult for a quadriplegic who has lost the use of the long tendons in his fingers, but it is easy for most other individuals.

There exist two classes of behavior which interest behavior modifiers—respondents and operants—discussed in Chapter 1. We have already described respondents (see Chapter 1 Section 1.2). Operants are usually voluntary behaviors affected by events that precede and follow them; this statement will be clarified shortly.

All the examples listed above (swimming, watching television, etc.) are operants. Other illustrations include using orthotic devices for grasping, paying attention, "sick talk," grooming, withdrawing from social contact, taking prescribed medications, colostomy care, or raising your hand in class to ask a question. (In the rest of this book, the word *behavior* will refer to *operant behavior*, except where indicated.)

Some activities are strong, and some are weak. Strength relates to how often behavior occurs—its *frequency*. Of all the ways to discuss the strength of behavior, frequency is the most valuable one for the nurse-practitioner. Very frequent behavior occurs many times; infrequent behavior occurs only a few times. To *accelerate* a behavior means to increase its frequency, and to *decelerate* it means to decrease its frequency.

The particular activities which the nurse wants to accelerate in the patient are the targets of treatment; they are *target behaviors*. Stating the goals of treatment or education in terms of various target behaviors avoids the problem of having objectives so broad that the techniques for obtaining them are unclear and undefined. For example, if one major objective in a program were to teach the patient to groom himself, the steps involved in attainment would become more apparent if they were listed as various target behaviors (e.g., bathing, combing hair, and brushing teeth), which constitute good grooming. Consider the goal of educating a competent nurse. Proficiency in the requisite behaviors that she must have in her repertoire requires that each activity become a target which nursing-school professors accelerate in their students.

A *stimulus* is any event impinging on or affecting an individual. *The environment*, which surrounds any individual, comprises stimuli. The sound of a plane, an itch, a nurse's uniform, a physician's office, the sight of a prosthetic device, the various tubes and wires connected to a patient on a coronary care unit, etc., are all stimuli.

Stimuli also may include the behaviors of other people. These behaviors are social stimuli, such as saying hello to a friend, which induces him to answer.

In addition, an individual's own activity may result in stimuli affecting his other behaviors. Thus, making an error while typing a term report is a behavior giving rise to stimuli which, in turn, are followed by the behavior of correcting the mistake.

The Effects of Stimuli on Behavior

Essentially, stimuli can affect behavior in five ways: Stimuli can have a neutral effect, an accelerating effect, a decelerating effect, a setting-the-occasion effect, or an eliciting effect. The eliciting effect has already been discussed in Chapter 1 in reference to respondent conditioning—stimuli can elicit involuntary activities. The following discussion illustrates the other four effects:

THE NEUTRAL EFFECT OF STIMULI. Stimuli that follow the occurrence of an activity may have no demonstrable effect on the frequency of the behavior. For example, if, while eating your dinner, you hear the sound of a plane in the distance, the noise may not, in any way, influence your eating speed or the likelihood that you will eat similar foods in the same situation at some future time.

THE ACCELERATING EFFECT OF STIMULI. Stimuli that follow the occurrence of a behavior can increase its frequency. That is, the behavior can be made to occur more often by manipulating the events that follow it. Thus, if you raise your hand in class and your teacher never calls on you, your hand raising will be infrequent. But, if your teacher begins to pay attention to you and allows you to speak when you raise your hand, your hand raising will become more frequent. Stimuli that follow behavior and that increase its frequency (that accelerate the behavior) are called *positive reinforcers*. Thus, if hand raising occurs more often during class because it is followed by teacher attention and by permission to speak, these consequences are positive reinforcers. As another example, suppose you have just purchased reading glasses and after wearing them once, you find that you can read more efficiently than before, that is, faster and for greater periods of time. You are likely to wear them again the next time you read and each time thereafter. The important consequences of wearing your glasses are that you can read faster and for greater periods of time.

But reading faster and for greater periods of time are positive reinforcers only because the behavior (wearing your glasses) followed by these stimulus events, increased. It is unwise to label a stimulus a positive reinforcer without first establishing that it accelerates the behavior it follows.

The nurse *cannot* assume that a stimulus is automatically going to function as a positive reinforcer for a patient's behavior simply because the stimulus appears to be a pleasant event (e.g., food, an enjoyable conversation). What may be a positive reinforcer for one individual's behavior may be a neutral stimulus for someone else's —preferences differ.

Increasing the frequency of behavior by employing Positive Reinforcement is the major subject of this chapter. But behavior also may be accelerated by *Negative Reinforcement*; that is, a behavior can be increased because it escapes or because it avoids some painful or unpleasant stimulus (see Section 3.7).

THE DECELERATING EFFECT OF STIMULI. Some events, if made to follow a specific behavior, will reduce its frequency. Thus, if wearing glasses resulted in headaches, you would soon put them away permanently and perhaps would search for a new pair. A headache is an unwelcome consequence that would reduce the behavior (wearing glasses) it followed (see Chapter 4).

THE SETTING-THE-OCCASION EFFECT OF STIMULI. Stimuli that *precede* behavior as well as stimuli that *follow* behavior are important in understanding and in implementing behavior modification techniques. *Stimuli that precede behavior control its occurrence by indicating when, where, or under what conditions the occurrence will be followed by a reinforcer.* These stimuli do not function as elicitors, which induce respondents. A bright light shined in your eye elicits pupil contraction. But a green traffic light at an intersection doesn't elicit street-crossing behavior. Rather, the green light sets the occasion for crossing the street—a behavior followed by a number of positive consequences. If walking to the opposite side of the street when the traffic light is green is followed by a number of positive reinforcers (crossing the street when the traffic light is red is likely to have drastic consequences), the green light can come to set the occasion for crossing the street; when the traffic light is green (a stimulus), the individual is more likely to cross the street (a behavior) than when this light is not green. Thus, stimuli that precede a behavior *followed by positive reinforcers* can come to have an effect on (control) whether the behavior will occur.

For example, a nurse who administers positive reinforcers to a mental patient when he greets her appropriately (e.g., she says hello) may eventually come to set the occasion for this greeting; when the patient sees this nurse, he will say hello. If other nurses never positively reinforce this patient for his appropriate greeting behavior, they will not experience this behavior—the patient will not greet them.

Instructions from a physician to a nurse concerning appropriate medications for the patient or instructions from a nurse to a patient concerning health care practices are a very important class of stimuli which set the occasion for specified behaviors. (Instructions tell a person what behaviors are to be performed and when.)

In sum, the most important effects stimuli can have on operant behavior are to accelerate or to decelerate it and to set the occasion for it. Acceleration and deceleration deal with stimuli that follow behavior (consequences) and the setting-the-occasion effect has to do with stimuli that precede behavior (antecedents). Depending on its relationship to an individual's behavior, any particular stimulus can have one or more of these functions.

Maximizing the Likelihood of Accelerating the Behavior Desired

As indicated, the frequency (strength) of any behavior can be changed by altering its consequences. Positive reinforcers are results that can increase the strength of the behavior they follow. Thus, if hand raising occurs more often because it is followed by teacher attention, this consequence—teacher attention—is a positive reinforcer.

In order to accelerate a behavior, the nurse must arrange the patient's environment so that positive reinforcers follow the patient's desirable activities—positive reinforcers are administered *only if* the behavior to be accelerated occurs. When she accomplishes this arrangement, the positive reinforcer can be considered *contingent on* the specific behavior, and acceleration of the target behavior becomes possible. Thus, the relationship between the target behavior and the stimulus following it should be a contingent one, with the target behavior, in effect, producing the positive reinforcer.

If the connection between behavior and the events following it is not purposely arranged in this manner—so the reinforcer follows the desired behavior only—it is unlikely that the desired behavior will become strong.

At times, the arrangement between behavior and its consequences may be dangerous. For example, rushing toward a psychotic child, clutching him, or hugging him *only* when he's being self-destructive (e.g., is banging his head) can accelerate this violent behavior; if you make these consequences contingent on the child's self-destructive acts, you may inadvertently increase them. Conversely, attending to the child and showing him concern when he is *not* harming himself can have the desirable effect of increasing these *non*-self-destructive activities. The therapeutic contingency is for desirable behavior—not for undesirable behavior—to produce positive reinforcers. In short, reinforcing a psychotic child by paying attention to him when he is engaging in extremely undesirable behavior and failing to reinforce him when he is not a problem may be a dangerous strategy. The child may become worse. Creating an environment of tender loving care without regard for the activities of the patient is not likely to foster the development of desirable behavior. When the patient is engaging in desirable behaviors, he should receive positive reinforcers so that the desirable behaviors will be strengthened. For patients in mental hospitals, the most humane approach to treatment is to provide them with the *basic necessities* and then to administer more than the minimum amount of positive reinforcers, contingent on desirable behaviors (Bandura, 1969).

In sum, the relationship between behavior and positive reinforcers should be a contingent one, planned purposely if the objectives of treatment will be attained.

Behavior and Stimuli Preceding It

In general, this section extends the information presented under the topic involving the setting-the-occasion effect of stimuli. An event can set the occasion for the occurrence of a behavior provided that the event consistently precedes the reinforced behavior.

If a green light consistently precedes crossing the street—this activity is reinforced by getting to the other side safely, as well as in other ways—the green light can come to set the occasion for crossing the street. The nurse, the hospital environment, and so on can become occasions on which specific behaviors of the patient result in reinforcement—these factors set the occasion for specific behaviors.

As discussed previously, the behavior of one person can be a stimulus (social stimulus) that sets the occasion for the behavior of another person. Thus, some of the patient's activities can set the occasion for specific activities of the nurse. For example, if a patient recently transferred from a coronary care unit evidences an irregular pulse, his nurse will likely request an EKG—the patient's irregular pulse is a cue (it sets the occasion) for the nurse to request (a behavior) an electrocardiogram. Similarly, the inattentive behavior of a school-aged child may lead a public health nurse to arrange a hearing examination for him.

The point is the following: Certain behaviors of the patient set the occasion for the observant nurse to recommend or to implement specific actions; recommending or implementing them are behaviors proven useful in the past for other patients. The nurse derives reinforcement when the patient is helped through her efforts. In short, behaviors of the patient (e.g., irregular pulse) set the occasion for specific behaviors of the nurse (e.g., requesting an EKG) that result in positive consequences.

Various events can set the occasion for various activities, which the following example (LeBow, Gelfand, and Dobson, 1970) shows. The patient, a middle-aged male, had acquired a respiratory problem while he was in a mental hospital. Some of the attending physicians believed that the difficulty—it took the form of a harsh, high-pitched inspiratory sound similar to the wheezing of an asthma patient—stemmed from a previous regimen of prescribed drugs (phenothiazines). Needless to say, this behavior was unpleasant for everyone in the patient's environment (e.g., other patients and ward nurses). Because the ward was crowded, treatment for this problem took place in a small room one floor below. Desirable behavior was defined as breathing normally—breathing without the wheezing sound. After several weeks of modification, the powerful effect of the treatment room on the patient's breathing behavior was evident. As soon as he entered the room, normal breathing occurred. But this effect took place only in the treatment room. Also, it did not seem to matter who was administering treatment procedures, since more than one individual had endeavored to help the patient. Evidently, the treatment room itself became a stimulus for normal breathing.

Events that regularly precede behavior followed by reinforcers can come to set the occasion for the occurrence of the behavior. In the absence of these happenings, the individual is unlikely to perform the activity. If the occurrence of a behavior is reinforced when these events are present and is not reinforced when they are absent, a *discrimination* will be formed—certain events will set the occasion for the behavior and others will not. A discrimination can be taught purposely.

Consider the discrimination a paraplegic forms as a result of bladder and bowel retraining. He learns to recognize cues from his body about voiding or about not voiding. Specific signs such as "goose pimples," "perspiration," and "a sense of fullness" can come to set the occasion for toileting, whereas other events do not (Tudor, 1970).

Generally, small children are positively reinforced with attention from their parents for saying "meow" when they see a cat, not when they see a dog. For a child, the sight of a cat sets the occasion for saying "meow," whereas the sight of a dog does not, because saying "meow" is reinforced only in the presence of the cat. The sight of a dog will set the occasion for other verbal behavior ("bowwow"). Thus, a discrimination between how cats and dogs sound is taught.

People and situations—a mother, for example, because she is associated with many different reinforcers for her child's many behaviors, or the nurse who administers reinforcers contingent on specific patient activities—can come to set the occasion for behavior and, thereby, can influence it. In short, the stimuli preceding behavior markedly affect it and must be considered in behavior modification.

The process of *generalization* describes another way that foregoing stimuli can influence behavior. To illustrate, consider once again the patient with the high-pitched respiratory sound. If other situations, in addition to the small room, had come to set the occasion for breathing normally, generalization would have occurred. Generalization means that various circumstances provide the opportunity for a specific behavior, along with the ones under which the behavior was reinforced. If a particular nurse positively reinforces a patient's greeting, for example, the sight of this nurse will occasion this behavior. If the patient also begins to greet other people, in addition to the specific nurse who reinforced his greeting, generalization will have occurred—the greeting will have become generalized to other people, none of whom were specifically involved in the reinforcement program.

In some sense, generalization indicates failure to discriminate (Bijou and Baer, 1961). But if generalization didn't occur, behavior modification would be slow and arduous; each of the patient's activities, which the nurse desired to accelerate, would need to be reinforced in numerous situations or in the presence of numerous people or at various times. Behavior modification, conducted in hospitals or in other settings, must have results that generalize to the patient's natural environment (e.g., his home, business, or school). Desirable behaviors accelerated in the hospital must continue to occur outside it (see Sections 3.5 and 3.6).

It is not only possible to make certain stimuli come to set the occasion for a behavior—to delimit the stimuli that can occasion behavior—but it is also possible to delimit the behaviors that will occur. That is, the discrimination process can involve both stimuli and behaviors. For example, the nurse can reinforce a retarded child for naming various objects after she has presented him with a picture of the various objects. He will gradually learn to name things correctly. For the child, the picture of the object will set the occasion for correctly naming it (a behavior), if positive reinforcers (e.g., candy) follow the naming. Some of the words the child utters will be clear, and others may be garbled. Clearly stating the names of objects can be increased (more precision in the behavior), however if the nurse reinforces more intelligible words when the pictures are shown and if she no longer reinforces garbled words. Gradually, the child will learn to speak more distinctly when he is given the pictures; object naming (the behavior) will become more precise (Acker et al., 1970).

Furthermore, it is possible not only for behavior to generalize to new situations but also for new activities, other than those specifically accelerated, to take place. For example, if some of the components of hygienic self-care are accelerated (e.g., bathing), other desirable and related behaviors, such as polishing one's shoes, also may increase in frequency even though they specifically are not accelerated. This result will be a meaningful one in a behavior modification program.

In conclusion, it is important to realize that generalization and discrimination can be advantageous or disadvantageous depending on the behaviors, the patients, and the situations with which the nurse is dealing. Consequently, generalization and discrimination should be planned for or avoided in a behavior modification program, and never should be left merely to chance.

The Positive Reinforcement Procedure

The *Positive Reinforcement procedure* can be used to accelerate activities. Its treatment definition is as follows:

Positive Reinforcement is a method for increasing the frequency of a desired behavior by presenting a pleasant event (e.g., offering candy, praise, or money), contingent on the occurrence of the behavior. The nurse must arrange the patient's environment so that the desirable behavior produces the positive reinforcer.

There exist three elements of this definition that should be emphasized. First, positive reinforcers are events that if made contingent on behavior, result in its acceleration. To say that an event is a positive reinforcer, the nurse must demonstrate that the frequency of a particular activity increases when followed by this consequence.

Second, a positive reinforcer for one person's behavior may not be a positive reinforcer for another person's behavior. Considering the patient an individual requires the realization that some of his reinforcers are distinctively his own. Finding reinforcers is an important responsibility of the nurse interested in using behavior modification. Interviews with the patient or with his friends and relatives concerning what he enjoys, observation of what he does, and the previous experience of the nurse are helpful in finding reinforcers.

Third, the relationship between the desired behavior and its consequence must be a *planned, contingent one*. The target behavior, in fact, must be the behavior that is reinforced, not some other activity.

Application 1. Health Teaching for a Well Child

The public health nurse who visits homes or the nurse who teaches groups of parents about hygiene will find the following example (Madsen, 1965) of the Positive Reinforcement procedure useful. By employing positive reinforcers, parents could accelerate rapid and nonstressful toileting in their young child. The author of the article described the child as follows:

> The child was a nineteen-month-old girl, the only child of parents who were both college graduates. The child was not suffering from any behavior problems, was normal to above average in development . . . and appeared to have been disciplined with relative consistency by parents who were in marked agreement on child-rearing practices. It was further ascertained that the mother had recently purchased a small toilet, had removed all restraining devices, and allowed the child to sit on the toilet whenever she so desired. While at the time of consultation the mother was placing the child on the toilet and remaining with her, there had been no successful eliminations. Despite a regular eight-ounce glass of orange juice at both nap-time and bedtime, the child had remained dry on a number of occasions. The frequency of "dry diapers after bed" was noticeably on the increase. However, while there was evidence of physiological readiness and a relatively permissive approach to the situation, the mother did mention that the child was beginning to react with crying and tears after two days of placing

her on the toilet about four times a day. The mother, in discussing the situation, was noticeably anxious and was anticipating nothing but unpleasant experiences until the child was trained.[1]

Dr. Madsen suggested to the parents that they positively reinforce the toileting behavior they desired to accelerate and that they instruct the child about the reinforcement program. The target behavior was successfully eliminating in the toilet. Being on the toilet was the occasion on which the child's eliminating would be reinforced, and reinforcement administration was contingent on the child's successfully eliminating in the toilet. This procedure is described below:

> It was decided that the most efficient method of training would be to give the child a candy reward whenever there was successful elimination. It was recommended that immediately after a dry diaper in the morning or after a nap the mother should place the child on the toilet, read to her or entertain her in some way, and allow her to leave the toilet when she so desired. During this time on the toilet, the mother or father was to tell the child that she would receive candy if she "went" on the toilet. Candy was withheld after failures, although the parents occasionally gave the child candy after meals and [at] other times during the day, but always without any connotation of reward.[2]

Notice that for the parents, a major stimulus setting the occasion for their placing the child on the toilet was finding a dry diaper. For the child, being placed on the toilet became the occasion on which elimination was reinforced. The course of the program and some additional features (i.e., being praised in addition to being given candy) are illustrated below:

> The program was started when the child was eighteen months, twenty-nine days old, and thirty days before a scheduled trip. The second training session on the toilet ended in success on that occasion, and thereafter the child . . . (1) was given a brand of candy especially desired (Kraft Caramels) immediately upon

---

[1]C. H. Madsen, Jr., "Positive reinforcement in the toilet training of a normal child: A case report," p. 305. From *Case Studies in Behavior Modification*, edited by Leonard P. Ullmann and Leonard Krasner. Copyright © 1965 by Holt, Rinehart, & Winston, Inc. Reprinted by permission of Holt, Rinehart & Winston, Inc.

[2]Ibid., pp. 305–306.

completion of urination or defecation and before she was removed from the toilet; (2) was lavishly praised by one or both of the parents present; (3) was told that when she "went" in the toilet candy would be forthcoming; and (4) was told that it would be very nice if she told her daddy or mommy when she had "to go." The fourth day the child made the comment, "Urinate a toto, get candy." The fifth day the child was allowed to ask her parents to take her to the toilet when she wanted (instead of being placed on the toilet by the parents) and there were two successful performances. The frequency of independent action increased, until on the twelfth day after the start of the program, the parents were satisfied that the child was trained. After the fifteenth day the reinforcements were given only if requested by the child. The trip occurred on schedule and although there were five days of driving at least eight hours a day in the car, there were no (toilet) accidents and the child made consistent use of a portable toilet. Sixty days after the start of the program the child's requests for candy had dropped to zero and she was using the bathroom on her own. On a follow-up after six months, it was found that only during an illness lasting one week, at age twenty-two months had there been any relapses. This setback had been minor and affected only defecation. The mother reinstituted the reinforcement procedure and promised the child a candy reward upon successful elimination in the proper place. During the week of retraining the reward was given only when specifically requested by the child. This procedure was successful and there were few problems during the week of retraining after which the program ceased.[3]

In sum, within a short period of time and with little stress for all concerned, the parents of a normal child were able to accelerate her appropriate toileting both at home and in other situations—the behavior generalized to new situations. Two additional points are worth emphasizing. First, the material reinforcement (candy), essential in the beginning of the program, was eventually replaced by other reinforcers more aligned with social practices; that is, "being mature," or being adult became the important consequences of appropriate toileting. Second, because the parents were educated in administering the training procedures, they were able to deal efficiently with a relapse; the mother reinstituted the previously suc-

---

[3]Ibid., p. 306.

cessful procedures. Both of these points will be discussed in Sections 3.5 and 3.6.

TERMS AND QUESTIONS

Terms

Behavior
Frequency of behavior
Accelerating behavior
Decelerating behavior
Target behavior
Stimuli
Environment
Positive reinforcer
Contingent relationship
Discrimination
Generalization
Setting-the-occasion effect of stimuli
Positive Reinforcement procedure

Questions

1. What are the advantages of formulating the goals of a behavior modification program in terms of target behaviors?
2. How can you ascertain if an event is a positive reinforcer?
3. What are setting-the-occasion and accelerating effects of stimuli on behavior? Contrast.
4. What does this statement mean? A purposely planned, contingent relationship should exist between behaviors and stimuli if the behaviors are to be accelerated.

3.2 *BENEFICIALLY IMPLEMENTING POSITIVE REINFORCEMENT: TYPES OF REINFORCERS*

This section deals with types of reinforcers that can be made contingent on desirable behavior.

Primary Reinforcers

Primary reinforcers are inborn—they are events that will accelerate the behavior they follow for almost everyone (e.g., air, water, food, rest, and sex).

The effectiveness of a consequence which can function as a reinforcer for an individual's behavior can vary; that is, the potency of reinforcers can change. *Deprivation* and *Satiation* are two processes affecting the potency of reinforcers. As indicated in Chapter 2, deprivation influences the potency of a reinforcer in this way: The more the individual is denied the reinforcer, within limits, the more powerful the reinforcer becomes—the more effective in accelerating behavior at a given time. Thus, an individual deprived of oxygen (primary reinforcer) will urgently engage in attempts to obtain it. The potency of oxygen as a primary reinforcer will depend on the extent to which an individual is deprived of it.

Satiation, in contrast, reduces the potency of a reinforcer. The more the individual is administered the reinforcer, the less influential it becomes in strengthening behavior at a given time. Thus, if an abundant supply of food is usually available at the dinner table, and an individual consumes the food until he is full (perhaps he eats more than enough), the food will temporarily lose its reinforcing potency, and behaviors that result in food—that have food as their consequence—will be unlikely to occur, until the person is hungry again. In short, Deprivation refers to being without the reinforcer, and Satiation refers to being given more than enough of it; generally, both Deprivation and Satiation are *temporary* processes. As time without the reinforcer increases, its potency is enhanced, but with repeated administrations of the reinforcer, its potency is reduced; these processes apply especially to primary reinforcers.

For some socially withdrawn retarded persons or for some mental patients, primary reinforcers (e.g., food) are extremely useful in the beginning stages of behavior modification. Other reinforcers, such as praise or attention from the nurse, may not be potent during these periods, and primary reinforcers must be employed to accelerate desirable behavior. As will be discussed, primary reinforcers administered in the early stages of behavior modification can be instrumental in making these other reinforcers potent.

Acquired Reinforcers

Acquired reinforcers are not inborn; they acquire the power to strengthen behavior sometime after birth. Varied events are acquired reinforcers—praise, attention, being loved, gaining approval, getting good grades in school, going home from the hospital, money, social interaction, being liked, being respected, and many more.

Events can become acquired reinforcers *if they are associated with the presentation of already potent reinforcers.* For example, if a bell signals lunch (rings immediately before lunch time), the bell can become an acquired reinforcer. Lunch time, the opportunity to eat, is a potent reinforcer. Because the sound of the bell regularly *precedes* eating—it sets the occasion for eating which is reinforced by food—the bell also will become a reinforcer. Once this process occurs, the sound of the bell will acquire the power to accelerate other activities, such as looking at your watch just before the bell is about to ring. Because the sound of the bell follows the behavior —looking at your watch—it will strengthen this behavior. The contingency between looking at your watch and the sound of the bell is not purposely arranged—it is accidental. Nevertheless, because the sound of the bell is a reinforcer that follows looking at your watch, this behavior will be strengthened. To reiterate, the bell will become an acquired reinforcer because it is associated with the administration of an already potent reinforcer, in this case, food.

Going home after a stay in the hospital is a pleasant event for most people. For others, notably for some mental patients, it is not a reinforcer. In order to prevent long-term hospitalization, the staff should try to make returning home or going to some other situation a positive event. Ayllon and Azrin (1968) made such an attempt with one female mental patient who resisted the idea of going to a half way house. She refused to be transferred there. The one time that she was placed in the half-way house she was soon rehospitalized. This reluctance to leave the mental hospital probably applied to her long stay there; many chronic mental patients do not want to leave the mental hospital. To help make going to the half-way house reinforcing, the authors exposed the patient to the reinforcers existing there; that is, the patient accompanied an attendant on visits to the half-way house, at which time she could observe former patients eating or engaging in other reinforcing activities. Through a *gradual* lengthening of the visits and through exposure of the patient to the potent reinforcers in the half-way house, going there acquired positive value. The patient requested to be discharged from the hospital to the half-way house after only six visits to it.

In essence, the new environment acquired reinforcing value for the patient. She was helped to make the transition gradually from the hospital to the half-way house; that is, she was helped to adjust to this new place.

For many individuals the transition from one environment to another may be accompanied by a period of uneasiness or apprehension. The severity of the patient's reaction to a sudden change in his surroundings—that is, how long and how much he feels upset—is related to both his previous experience with such abrupt changes and the attempts made to re-orientate him. For many, leaving the everyday natural environment to enter the hospital or transferring from the hospital to some other treatment situation is particularly frightening and uncomfortable. Since behavior modification, which may be necessary in the new environment, is hindered if the patient is fearful, the nurse should attempt to make him more comfortable. A discussion with adult patients pertaining to the specific behaviors sought (e.g., detailing the reinforceable behaviors for mental patients new on a psychiatric ward) can reduce their initial uneasiness. With children, the nurse specifically may have to establish herself as a source of positive reinforcement by freely administering positive reinforcers (e.g., praise or candy). In this way, she can help to reduce a child's uneasiness in a "different" environment (e.g., a doctor's office or a hospital ward). Although administering of positive reinforcers should not follow flagrantly unadaptive behavior, they should be made readily available during this stage for minimally desirable behavior.

Events that can function as acquired reinforcers—reinforcers accelerating behavior which they follow—also can function as stimuli setting the occasion for other behavior, followed by other reinforcers. In fact, once a stimulus sets the occasion for behavior, it is likely to become an acquired reinforcer. Thus, the sound of the bell will set the occasion for eating, and it also will reinforce looking at the watch. A nurse can set the occasion for a patient's behavior as well as reinforce it.

More specifically, the nurse's presence and approval can offer the opportunity for some of the patient's behaviors—the nurse's presence and approval *precede* certain activities of the patient. And, the nurse's presence and approval can function as a reinforcer for some of the patient's behavior—the nurse's presence and approval follow certain activities of the patient.

For example, giving the patient a bath can be an event that communicates caring (Davis, 1970); it is pleasant for the patient. Because it is a reinforcing activity for the bed patient, the association of the nurse with this activity results in her presence becoming an event setting the occasion for behaviors of the patient that result in the bath. That is, when the nurse is present, the bath (reinforcer) is likely to follow various behaviors of the patient such as requesting a bath, acting friendly, or even resting silently. *The nurse's presence, conversation, attention, and approval, in short, make reinforc-*

ing events such as the bath possible. Once the nurse's presence, conversation, attention, and approval acquire this setting-the-occasion function the nurse, herself, also very likely will acquire reinforcing potency. More specifically, attention and approval from the nurse will become potent reinforcers capable of accelerating various behaviors of the patient. If made contingent on the patient's listening and on his demonstrating comprehension of various home-care instructions, these consequences—attention and approval from the nurse—will facilitate teaching.

Many nursing activities will result in the nurse's presence, for example, becoming a stimulus which can both set the occasion and can reinforce various behaviors. The acquired reinforcing value of the nurse can be potent in accelerating many desirable patient behaviors. Although the nurse may not need to establish herself independently as a reinforcer for all patients in order to teach, for some patients who seem unresponsive to social approval, this process may be necessary.

Generalized-Acquired Reinforcers

Some acquired reinforcers are extremely potent. They can be used to strengthen a wide variety of behaviors. Money, attention, and praise are potent reinforcers because more than one source of deprivation affects them. For example, possessing money makes possible the acquisition of such diverse events as food, shelter, good clothes, weekend activities, and automobiles. Money can be used as a reinforcer almost indefinitely as long as it can enable someone to buy something. But food, a primary reinforcer, will only be potent as long as the individual is hungry. In addition, bell ringing, an acquired reinforcer, will only remain a potent reinforcer as long as lunch follows it. *Both food and bell ringing are tied to one source of deprivation. Money, on the other hand, is tied to various sources of deprivation.* Acquired reinforcers affected by many sources of deprivation (e.g., money, praise, and attention) are called *generalized-acquired reinforcers.*

Generalized-acquired reinforcers will remain potent longer than primary and other acquired ones, such as the sound of the bell. Yet, if having money no longer leads to many of the pleasures in life, money would lose its effectiveness as a reinforcer. For example, confederate currency is not a reinforcer for most people. Similarly, if you were lost in the Mojave desert while you were carrying a 50-pound sack of $100 bills, it is conceivable that lightening your load would be more attractive than keeping the money. The point is the following: Only rarely will a generalized-acquired reinforcer diminish in potency, but it is possible.

Money in the form of tokens has been employed as a potent generalized-acquired reinforcer in various situations (see Chapter 7). The token becomes a powerful reinforcer because it can be used to buy various other reinforcers. Praise and attention from others also are potent generalized-acquired reinforcers for most individuals and are useful in rehabilitating mental patients, in treating disabled individuals, or in health teaching to families and large groups.

For some people (e.g., some mental patients and retarded individuals), praise and attention from others or even money (tokens) have either ceased or never have become reinforcers. Developing desirable behavior in these patients requires using primary reinforcers (e.g., food). One goal, however, should be to help convert these types of consequences, especially praise and attention from others, *into* potent reinforcers. This change can be accomplished by coupling praise from the nurse with primary reinforcers. When praise from the nurse becomes associated with the delivery of primary reinforcers (e.g., food), then praise from the nurse can become a reinforcer employed to accelerate numerous desirable behaviors for many individuals. Increasing the potency of praise and attention—they are social reinforcers—can be a crucial step in producing lasting behavior changes, that is, durable changes. Social reinforcers, made contingent on many desirable behaviors by the outside community, can be instrumental in making behavior modification meaningful (see Section 3.5).

Apart from the advantages of increasing the potency of reinforcers found in the natural environment, using generalized-acquired reinforcers in behavior modification programs is encouraged for the following technical reasons:

(1) *Satiation will not take place quickly because more than one major source of deprivation affects the power of the generalized-acquired reinforcer.* In order for food (a primary reinforcer) to become a potent reinforcer, the individual must be deprived of food. For rest to become a potent reinforcer, the individual must lack rest. Deprivation of food will not markedly affect the potency of rest as a reinforcer or vice-versa. The effective condition of deprivation, with primary reinforcers especially, is tied to the *one* reinforcer being used in the behavior modification program, not to some other reinforcer. In general, if a reinforcer is affected by only one source of deprivation, it will lose its potency faster with repeated administrations, than if it is affected by several sources of deprivation. Thus,

food temporarily will become ineffective as a reinforcer as soon as the individual has had enough to eat; but reinforcers such as money and praise, affected by many deprivations, will remain potent almost indefinitely. Because money buys so many primary and other types of tangible reinforcers, and since both money and praise, for many individuals, are important precursors to obtaining high status (non-tangible reinforcers) their potency rarely diminishes.

(2) *Using generalized-acquired reinforcers does not delay the progress of any one treatment session.* Tokens, for instance, can be delivered to the patient immediately after the performance of the desirable behavior and can be cashed in for other reinforcers at a later time. On the other hand, delivering an edible primary reinforcer, such as food, following the desirable behavior and immediately consuming it can slow down the treatment session. This problem can be avoided, to some extent, by not allowing the patient to expend the reinforcer immediately. The reinforcers can be stored in some convenient container (in full view of the patient) after their administration, or the patient can be allowed to consume the edibles immediately after their delivery, if they are presented in very small portions (e.g., a bit of candy).

In conclusion, it is important to emphasize that combining reinforcers is advantageous. In particular, mixing primary and generalized-acquired reinforcers, such as food and praise, or mixing two generalized-acquired reinforcers, such as tokens and praise, are valuable strategies. When possible, using several reinforcers in any one program is advisable.

Activity Reinforcers (Personalized Reinforcers)

People vary. One person's tastes differ from another's. What can you do to help a patient behave more capably, if he tells you (or if you notice) that he doesn't want anything? The answer to this frequent question is to *observe what the patient does and to make this activity a reinforcer.* Any activity that an individual frequently performs can function as a reinforcer and, therefore, can be used to accelerate desirable behavior (Premack, 1963); that is, *behaviors* which a person enjoys doing can be used as reinforcers for accelerating other ones. Even what appears to be doing nothing, if examined closely by the nurse, may be an activity. Thus, sitting on a chair and doing nothing can be used as a reinforcer if it occurs frequently. When the opportunity to sit on a chair for a specified period is made contingent on the performance of some desirable behavior, the desirable behavior can be accelerated.

Activities such as going on a weekend pass for mental patients, free-time for deaf children (Osborne, 1969), taking driving lessons for adolescents, finger painting for children, listening to favorite music for geriatric patients, having supervisory responsibilities for narcotics patients, helping other alcoholics for alcoholic patients, participating in decisions for welfare recipients, discussing infant care with the nurse for expectant parents, and talking about dietary and other health-care practices with the nurse for families and groups in ghetto areas are but a few of the many possible reinforcers. Regardless of the particular individual or group with whom the nurse is working, reinforcers are available. They may be very personalized—may be tailored to each individual's preferences.

The major problem with activity reinforcers is that they cannot be administered contingent on *each* occurrence of the desirable behavior, because if they were, treatment would be delayed inordinately and, in addition, the patient would probably tire of the activity. One useful solution is for the nurse to employ generalized-acquired reinforcers, such as tokens, as a medium of exchange for the opportunity to engage in these other activity reinforcers. After earning tokens for engaging in desirable behavior, the patient can spend them on preferred activities.

This, of course, requires that some of the preferred activities be made unavailable until the patient engages in enough desirable behavior. It seems wiser to foster desirable behavior in a patient through carefully implementing preferred activities—controlled administration—than to allow him simply to engage in these activities, regardless of his behavior. If desirable behavior can be accelerated by using preferred activities, then it is unreasonable and not in the best interest of the patient to permit uncontrolled access to these reinforcers.

Watching what the individual does simplifies the problem of finding effective reinforcers. Everyone has reinforcers and these reinforcers can be discovered by careful observation (see Section 3.1 and Chapter 5). The nurse must recognize that reinforcers vary for different individuals and for the same individual at different times. Watching T.V. may be a preferred activity for a patient only during specified times during the day. Another patient may want to listen to music rather than to watch T.V. Effective behavior modification programs capitalize on the variety and the personalized qualities of available reinforcers.

In sum, there are several types of reinforcers available for the nurse to apply in behavior modification—food, tokens, attention, the opportunity to engage in preferred activities, and so on. Effective programs utilize potent reinforcers that resist satiation. Food may be used initially with individuals who do not respond to generalized-acquired reinforcers (e.g., approval or tokens). A goal when using food should be to enhance the effectiveness of generalized-acquired reinforcers. Also, a useful strategy in behavior modification is to strengthen desirable behavior with tokens, later redeemable for favored activities.

Application 2. Using a Generalized-Acquired Reinforcer for the Social Rehabilitation of a Mentally Disturbed Person

This case study (Kennedy, 1964)[4] shows how a generalized-acquired reinforcer, social approval, was used to help a man plagued with hallucinations, delusions, decreased productivity at work, and problems in living with his wife and two children. The potency of social approval and disapproval as consequences to behavior is made clear; the rapidity with which this patient was helped attests to this potency. The durability of the positive effects of treatment also provides evidence that, to be meaningful, behavior modification programs should attempt to use reinforcers found in the natural environment—social approval and attention. The nurses in this case study maintained the positive effects begun in therapy. This technique is a vital step toward rehabilitation. If a mental patient undergoing behavior modification spends the majority of his time on a psychiatric ward, where reinforcers are not administered on a desirable-behavior-contingent basis, the positive effects of behavior modification will be short lived. Psychiatric nurses have direct access to the patient and, consequently, can be purveyors of effective and durable treatment.

The patient, in the study below, was a 32-year-old insurance salesman who evidenced problems (e.g., hallucinations and delusions) that resulted in his being placed in a mental hospital. As described by the author:

> He was convinced that his life was intimately bound up with his own insurance policies and by omitting a payment on his insurance premium he had lost part of himself. He had shown evi-

---

[4]Trudy Kennedy, "Treatment of chronic schizophrenia by behaviour therapy: Case reports," *Behaviour Research and Therapy*, 2, 1964, 1–6.

> dence of decreased work efficiency and began to drink heavily. His appetite and sleeping habits were poor. His wife reported increasing abruptness and irritability in his treatment of her and the two children.[5]

To help this patient, the target behavior of coherent and relevant speech was selected. The positive reinforcer employed by the therapist and the ward nurses was social approval. This potent reinforcer was made contingent on the occurrence of the target behavior. In addition, social disapproval was made contingent on inappropriate speech. This latter technique was employed to decelerate undesired verbal behavior (see Chapter 4). The procedures and the results were recorded as follows:

> This patient was seen for half-an-hour interviews on a three times a week basis. He was started on psychotropic medications, 300 mg chlorpromazine daily, which was later reduced to 100 mg daily. The first interviews were primarily to obtain an adequate factual history and to attempt to gain the confidence of the patient. The therapist gave no indication of consistent approval or disapproval of any statements made by the patient. During the second week of treatment, each frankly delusional statement was objected to by the therapist, using both verbal and nonverbal (i.e., facial expression) cues of disapproval. Facts known to the therapist were brought forward as objections to delusional statements. The therapist insisted that the patient speak of problems concerning his job and family relationships and by so doing he gained the attention and presumably approval of the therapist. A gradual change in his speech content developed and each demonstration of change to a more reality-oriented approach to problems was strongly reinforced both by the therapist's attitude and by direct expression of approval. This attitude was continued in the general ward routine by the nursing staff, who verbalized their approval and appreciation of his modified speech and behavior. He was elected ward president and this in itself was a reinforcement of his changed behavior. Towards the end of his stay in the hospital he was able to continue studying for his examinations as a chartered life underwriter. Such studying was reinforced by permitting him to remain in his room. Since leaving the hospital, he has been seen at monthly intervals by another therapist. His first follow-up assess-

---

[5]Ibid., p. 1.

ment was conducted eight weeks after his discharge. At this time he was working full-time and his wife stated that he was more tolerant of her and the children. Sessions since then have been fifteen minutes in duration and entirely devoted to discussion of practical matters concerning his job and home life. He does not bring forward any delusional ideas and is functioning well in a responsible job as an insurance sales manager, with six to eight men working in subordinate positions. His stay in the hospital was less than three months.[6]

Application 3. Using Verbal Reinforcers to Accelerate Wheelchair Pushing for a Patient with Parkinson's Disease

Although the behavior accelerated in this study (Goodkin, 1966)[7] was not as crucial to the patient's recovery as the one discussed in the previous example, its modification does attest to the general usefulness of verbal consequences in ameliorating various activities. Goodkin described the patient as follows:

> Mrs. B. is a 61-yr-old woman with a 15-yr history of Parkinson's disease. It was called to [the experimenter's] attention by the psychologist working with Mrs. B. and by the activities of the daily living therapist working with her that Mrs. B. refused to push her wheelchair. Mrs. B. stated that it was no use trying because even very small children were able to propel their chair much faster than she was. It was suggested by her physician that it would be advisable for Mrs. B. to propel her own chair because it would make her less dependent on others. Moreover, muscle tests suggested that she did have the strength and range of motion to perform the activity.
>
> Observations of the patient in her regular activities in the daily living class suggested that she had put forth very little effort in propelling her wheelchair and that she spent nearly half of the session complaining to the therapist that she could not do it.[8]

After observing this patient's behavior, the author of the study began treatment. To accelerate wheelchair pushing, he designated

---

[6]Ibid., p. 2.

[7]R. Goodkin, "Case studies in behavioral research in rehabilitation," *Perceptual and Motor Skills*, 23, 1966, 171–182. Reprinted with permission of author and publisher.

[8]Ibid., p. 175.

the reinforceable behavior (e.g., moving the wheelchair five feet), the reinforcers, and the measure of the effectiveness of treatment (time). The procedures and results of three days are described below:

> Mrs. B. was seen by (the experimenter) in a classroom free from distractions of other people. Prior to the introduction of the experimental conditions, strips of red tape were placed on the floor to mark off each 5-ft interval of a 20-ft distance. Each trial consisted of having the patient move 5 ft. . . . There were 1-min rest intervals before starting each new trial. The average time to propel the chair 5 ft was calculated at the end of each session. The patient was seen for approximately 20 min each day.
>
> The treatment started on the second day. It consisted of: (1) telling Mrs. B. that she was doing well, (2) telling her the number of seconds it took her to go 5 ft, and (3) telling her how many seconds she cut off her previous record when she performed faster. When she performed more slowly, she was told nothing. Each day the patient received her initial verbal reinforcement after her first response that excelled her average time of the previous day.
>
> At the end of the session the patient was told her average time for that day, and it was compared with that obtained on previous days. In this way she tended to speak more about her own performance and less of how she compared with others. She also complained very little during the second and third sessions . . . Each day she spontaneously asked to do more trials. Mrs. B. wheeled her chair faster and further each day. Unfortunately she was unable to continue with this procedure because of her discharge from the Institute.[9]

Several aspects of this study should be clarified. First, because a combination of reinforcers was employed, it was difficult to evaluate which reinforcer was crucial or whether the combination per se was necessary (see Chapter 5). This disadvantage of employing several reinforcers, however, was offset somewhat by the increased likelihood that one of the reinforcers used remained potent. By employing several reinforcers at once or by varying them, the nurse can reduce the risk that all the reinforcers will lose their strengthening properties. An efficient approach for maintaining the availability of potent reinforcers in a behavior modification program is to

---

[9]Ibid., pp. 175–176.

create a *reinforcer menu*, on which various reinforcers are pictured or listed (Addison and Homme, 1966). The patient can choose the most potent reinforcer on the menu at any given time or, if necessary, the nurse can determine the most influential one for the patient.

Second, by informing the patient about the amount of time it took her to move her wheelchair five feet and how much improvement she had made (reinforcers 2 and 3), the author gave her feedback concerning her progress; feedback (i.e., the patient is informed about his behavior changing in the desired direction) is an important consequence that may be used to accelerate behavior.

Third, to measure the change in the target behavior (wheelchair pushing), the speed with which the patient propelled her chair was calculated. Frequency of behavior was not used as the measure of behavior change in this study. Frequency, however, could have been employed as a measure of the number of instances the patient, unassisted, propelled her wheelchair outside of the treatment situation. This method would have indicated if the effects of treatment generalized.

Application 4. A Technique for Managing Unruly Behavior in Well Children

Healthy young children perform many bothersome activities that adults find disturbing. Consequently, working with young children may be a trying experience for anyone. In the next study (Homme et al., 1963),[10] desirable behavior was accelerated in a group of young nursery school children by using tokens and activity reinforcers. The authors of the report observed that often the children would not obey the instruction to sit in their chairs. Instead, they would perform a variety of activities such as, "screaming, running around the room, pushing chairs," and so forth. Because these behaviors occurred frequently, they were designated activity reinforcers. (Any behavior, as indicated, that occurs frequently can function as an activity reinforcer.) To accelerate desired behavior (e.g., sitting quietly) and to avoid using any punishment, the authors allowed the children to be *noisy*. But they made this activity contingent on desirable behaviors. Thus, at times, when the children were quiet, a bell was rung and they were told to "run and scream." After another signal, the children were instructed, for example, to

[10]L. E. Homme, P. C. deBaca, J. V. Devine, R. Steinhorst, and E. J. Rickert, "Use of the Premack principle in controlling the behavior of nursery school children," *Journal of the Experimental Analysis of Behavior*, 6, 1963, 544.

sit down. Later in the study, they were given tokens, contingent on desirable behavior; the tokens were redeemable for the opportunity to perform preferred activities. Thus, with a simple and painless manipulation, control over the children's unruly behaviors was quickly achieved.

This classic study was originally published as an illustration of the ease with which desirable behaviors can be accelerated simply by making the opportunity to engage in preferred activities contingent on them. Tokens are convenient in these studies because they can be given immediately following the desirable behavior and can be cashed in later for the preferred activity. Immediate reinforcement is important (see Section 3.3).

Activity reinforcers have been used frequently to accelerate desirable behavior and are applicable to a variety of problems. For example, if the nurse is confronted with a child who refuses to take the medications prescribed for him while he is at home, this problem may be resolved by constructing a behavioral agreement between the child and his parents or the nurse which incorporates activity reinforcers. A *behavioral agreement* or *contract* is a device that specifically designates activities to be performed and contingent reinforcers to be delivered. A behavioral contract clearly specifies its terms. Thus, if the child followed the prescribed medical regimen (e.g., if he took medications on time, ate designated foods, and performed designated exercises) he could earn tokens toward the purchase of preferred activities listed in the contract. The parents or nurse must agree to redeem the tokens on demand, when the child lives up to his part of the agreement. The preferred activities, their cost, and the amount payable for the occurrence of each desirable behavior must be clearly specified (written down) for the contract to work. At first glance, this technique may seem like bribery. But bribery, as indicated previously, refers to payment for corrupt behavior. Following a medical regimen is certainly not behaving corruptly. And using positive reinforcers to accelerate desirable behaviors such as these is not bribery.

Consider this example which incorporated a behavioral contract for helping a family improve the relationship among its members (Coe, 1970). Its problems were centered around the 12-year-old son. To specify the important behaviors and reinforcers for the boy, three lists of activities were constructed by the family. The first depicted behaviors which the boy did, but shouldn't do (don'ts). The second included behaviors which the boy should do, but didn't (do's) and the third consisted of activities the child enjoyed (activity reinforcers). All the family members agreed on the contents of each list and a behavioral contract was established. The boy was positively reinforced with tokens for behaviors on the "do" list and was charged for behaviors on the "don't" list as well as for activity reinforcers. Thus, a successful financial plan was carefully constructed with income and costs balancing.

For various problems, especially those involving families with well children, the nurse can employ behavioral contracts that utilize activity reinforcers. An agreement can result in rapid improvement of behavior without undue stress for anyone involved. Teaching behavior principles, such as these, to families is a strategy of prevention which the nurse can efficiently utilize (see Section 3.6).

TERMS AND QUESTIONS

Terms

Satiation
Primary reinforcers
Acquired reinforcers
Generalized-acquired reinforcers
Activity reinforcers
Reinforcer menu
Behavioral contract

Questions

1. How may primary reinforcers be used to develop the potency of social reinforcers (e.g., praise)?
2. What is the crucial difference between primary and acquired reinforcers?
3. What is the crucial difference between acquired reinforcers and generalized-acquired reinforcers?
4. How may you effectively combine generalized-acquired reinforcers (tokens) with activity reinforcers?
5. How will you establish yourself as a positive reinforcer for a socially isolated adult?
6. How will you use a behavioral contract to design a program for helping a crippled child to perform his exercises?

3.3 *BENEFICIALLY IMPLEMENTING POSITIVE REINFORCEMENT: ADMINISTERING REINFORCERS*

The effectiveness of behavior modification is related not only to the validity of its principles, but also to the efficiency of its implementation. The difference between successful and unsuccessful outcomes often is directly related to how the procedures are applied. A thorough understanding of the ways of efficiently implementing behavior modification procedures will separate the successful behavior modifier from the unsuccessful one. Many parents or teachers who do not understand the intricacies of behavior changing procedures claim that they already have tried behavior modification and that it doesn't work. Undoubtedly, we all have experienced success and failure at behavior modification. More specifically, we have been both successful and unsuccessful in changing our own behavior and the behavior of others when we have either purposely or unwittingly applied modification principles. Similarly, our parents express success and failure in their attempts to mold our behavior. These inconsistent results reflect many issues, particularly those concerning the efficient administration of behavior principles. This section is addressed to the issues concerning the efficient administration of positive reinforcers.

Administer Potent Reinforcers

The necessity of using potent reinforcers has already been discussed. To reiterate briefly, the more powerful the consequences of behavior, the greater the likelihood that the behavior will be successfully accelerated. The most potent reinforcers—reinforcers which do not easily lose their power to reinforce—are generalized-acquired (e.g., praise, attention, tokens). Preferred activities, in addition, are potent reinforcers which can be used in various situations and which easily can be combined with tokens.

Administer Reinforcers Contingent on Behavior

This issue also, has already been discussed. The occurrence of the behavior to be accelerated should produce the reinforcer. The relationship, therefore, between the behavior and its consequence—the positive reinforcer—must be arranged purposely so that the behavior results in the positive reinforcer.

Administer Reinforcers Consistently

The most efficient way to strengthen behavior is to reinforce it whenever it occurs. Initially, therefore, *every* occurrence of the behavior should be followed by delivery of the reinforcer.

The frequency with which reinforcers are administered (how often reinforcers are given) is related to what is called the schedule of reinforcement. In this book, we will consider three schedules of reinforcement. Two of them, which will be discussed in Section 3.5, are useful in making the behavior modification results durable.

If a reinforcer is administered following *each* occurrence of the specified desirable behavior, the schedule of reinforcement is *continuous*; that is, *reinforcement occurs 100% of the time.* Whenever the behavior occurs, the reinforcer follows. A *continuous reinforcement schedule*—each occurrence of the target behavior is reinforced—should be employed in the modification program until the behavior to be accelerated becomes strong.

For instance in Application 1 (the toilet-training example), each time the child successfully eliminated in the toilet, she was given a candy and was praised. This continuous schedule of reinforcement was in operation until the target behavior (successful elimination in the toilet) became strong.

Administer Reinforcers Immediately

Do not be tardy in administering reinforcers. More specifically, they should be delivered *immediately* after a behavior occurs if it is to be accelerated. Thus, the administration of reinforcers should be prompt. If they are delayed, a possibility exists that a behavior other than the one specifically designated will be accelerated. For example, if you want to strengthen a six-month-old child's laughing, it is more effective to pick him up or to hug him immediately after he has laughed than to do so five minutes later, when he may be chewing on a toy or may be waving his arms. Administering reinforcers at this time would probably strengthen these other behaviors, not laughing.

To correct a quadraplegic patient's use of an Electric Torque Motor (Trombly, 1966), a device employed for opening and closing fingers, you should provide him with immediate feedback, not feedback 15 minutes later, during a discussion.

Similarly, helping total-nursing-care patients with multiple physical handicaps to develop motor skills necessitates immediate reinforcement (Rice, McDaniel, and Denney 1968).

In education, teaching machines have proven useful, in part, because immediate reinforcement follows correct answers. Immediate reinforcement is more effective than delayed reinforcement in terms of progress with educational material. Thus, teaching the coronary patient about diet, drugs, and general home-care practices (Hahn and Dolan, 1970) while he is in a rehabilitation unit can be effectively carried out if the patient's and his family's understanding of the physician's directives is reinforced immediately. Before the patient returns home, his knowledge as well as his family's knowledge of the physician's instructions should be queried by the nurse, and accurate verbalizations should be immediately reinforced. Praise or affirmation from the nurse that the patient and his family are correct may serve as reinforcers.

In group education situations, such as teaching several arthritic patients about arthritis (Valentine, 1970), immediate feedback may be arranged by making written answers to any test available directly following a patient's completion of the test. This technique is efficient for correcting errors.

It is possible to learn even though reinforcers are delayed (e.g., course grades are given at the end of a term), but this strategy is not necessarily the most productive one. Adult patients with various problems can be told that reinforcers will follow their desirable behaviors at some later time; that is, the interval between the occurrence of a behavior and the administration of a reinforcer may be relatively long. A reinforcer may be made contingent on the occurrence of a behavior and still may be administered after a relatively long time, provided that the patient understands the contingency—that he knows the designated behavior will lead to the administration of the favored consequence, at some later time.

The most efficient way to reinforce a behavior (to teach a new behavior or to accelerate an infrequent one) for many patients, however, is to reinforce it immediately. If the most potent reinforcer for a patient is a preferred activity, the interval between the occurrence of a certain number of desirable behaviors and the administration of this activity reinforcer may be bridged by promptly following each desired behavior with a token. For example, if a retarded child correctly uses or clearly names some object (the nurse having designated that these are desirable behaviors), a token may be given immediately after the behavior occurs. Once a specific number of tokens have been earned, they may be cashed in for the preferred reinforcer (e.g., extra playtime). Thus, acquired reinforcers (tokens) may be used to overcome the delay between the occurrence of desirable behaviors and the administration of a preferred reinforcer.

Even if a patient is simply told that he is correct—is given verbal feedback about his behavior—this is best presented immediately following his behavior.

Administer Enough Reinforcers

The quantity of reinforcement, that is, the number of reinforcers administered following a behavior affects the results of a behavior modification program. Both too much and too little reinforcement may lead to poor results—the target behavior may not be strengthened.

Thus, if too much reinforcement follows the occurrence of the target behavior, the reinforcer-administrator may run out of reinforcers or the reinforcer-recipient may stop performing the desirable behavior because he has accumulated *enough* reinforcers (i.e., he is no longer deprived; he is satiated).

For example, suppose a father wants his 15-year-old son, a high school junior, to improve his grades. After analyzing the components of receiving good marks, the father may decide to reinforce his son's study behavior. Suppose, however, the father uses $100 as the reinforcer. The contingency between the behavior and the reinforcer is one hour of study results in $100. The result of this approach is likely to be bankruptcy; that is, the father will soon run out of reinforcers.

Another approach that will avoid bankruptcy is to use car privileges as a reinforcer. If the father, however, administers this reinforcer in excessive amounts (e.g., seven hours of driving the car for one hour of study), it may rapidly lose its potency. The son may earn so many hours of driving time with so few hours of study that he will soon stop studying. The effects of both of these approaches will be the same: studying will remain a weak behavior.

On the other hand, if too little reinforcement is made contingent on a behavior, the behavior still will remain unaccelerated. Although the reinforcer-administrator will remain solvent, and the reinforcer-recipient will not be overly reinforced, the behavior, nevertheless, will remain weak. Suppose, for example, the father in the illustration above reinforces each study hour with one cent. This paucity of reinforcement will not lead to intense studying; that is, the son will give up studying because it doesn't pay off. And the studying behavior will remain unaccelerated.

Until the son can derive satisfaction from the behavior itself (see Concluding Statement), engaging in the desirable behavior (studying) has to be worth his effort. Enough reinforcement must occur.

For the nurse-practitioner, a balanced amount of reinforcement means using enough reinforcement to accelerate the behavior but not so much that the patient loses interest in performing it or so much that the nurse runs out of reinforcers. Thus, in the initial phase of a behavior modification program, the amount of reinforcement following each occurrence may be on the plentiful side; but as the behavior shows evidence of strengthening, the amount of reinforcement should be gradually reduced (see Section 3.5). Recording the frequency of behavior (see Chapter 5) will help the nurse decide when and how much to reduce the quantity of reinforcement.

Administer Reinforcers Sincerely

It is essential that the nurse who administers positive reinforcers, such as the word "good," following a behavior do so sincerely. Different individuals have different communication styles. But all behavior modifiers have to be consistent in what they communicate. To say "good" halfheartedly or to exaggerate and to appear phony, for example, may be perceived by a patient as an ineffectual or perhaps as a punishing consequence.

Verbal reinforcers—social reinforcers—should be stated sincerely to maximize their effectiveness. Similarly, to say no to a retarded child in a weak and passive manner may not have the same effect on the behavior it follows as does a firm no—a no that means no.

As indicated in Chapter 2, civility, courtesy, and regard for the patient are just some of the essential behaviors or qualities of the nurse, which, apart from accurately administering reinforcers, can markedly affect the patient's behavior. For example, nonverbal communication (e.g., facial expressions) is important in conveying liking and regard or its opposite to the patient (Mehrabian, 1970). These types of event can affect the behavior modification program.

TERMS AND QUESTIONS

Terms

Continuous reinforcement schedule

Questions

1. With what type of patient would you expect immediate reinforcement, rather than delayed reinforcement, to be essential?
2. When were you lax in an important activity because you received too little reinforcement for engaging in it? Also, when were you lax in an important activity because you received too much reinforcement?

3.4 *BENEFICIALLY IMPLEMENTING POSITIVE REINFORCEMENT: PRODUCING BEHAVIOR*

To accelerate a behavior by administering positive reinforcers requires that it occur in order to be reinforced. For many patients, however, the desirable behavior the nurse wants to accelerate rarely or never occurs. The retarded child does not automatically feed or groom himself; the physically handicapped patient does not spontaneously perform the necessary health exercises; the immobile catatonic schizophrenic is unlikely just to begin to speak after years of being silent; the arthritic patient rarely performs, without being specifically taught, the important health care practices; and most delinquents do not suddenly become good students. These behaviors have to be built; that is, they have to be produced initially, before they can be reinforced.

The various procedures for producing behavior so that it can be strengthened is the subject of this section. These techniques are vital for individuals who rarely, if ever, perform the specific target behavior in question. In other words, to successfully implement the Positive Reinforcement procedure, the target behavior must be made to occur.

The procedures that will be discussed in this section may be employed in the following circumstances: where a new behavior is to be accelerated; where an old behavior which appears to be lost is to be reinstated (e.g., functional blindness); where the complexity of behavior is to be increased (e.g., teaching a patient about self-care for his illness or teaching general health-care practices); or where the nurse wants to accelerate a very infrequent behavior but cannot simply wait for it to occur so that it may be reinforced.

Shaping Behavior

Children do not learn spontaneously to speak English. The babbling sounds of an infant are molded gradually into normal speech. For example, when a child makes the sound *ah,* which approximates *Mom,* his parents usually are delighted and may hug or praise him; that is, when a child prattles a sound like the English word *Mom,* his parents are likely to reinforce him positively. At some point, he may babble an *M* sound resulting in *Mah,* and this increased approximation may also lead to reinforcement. The parents then raise the requirement for reinforcement and no longer encourage the child for an *ah* sound alone but, instead, demand the *Mah* sounds. By raising the requirement for reinforcement in this fashion, the parents gradually will mold *Mah* into *Mom.* Eventually, the child will be reinforced only if he says a clear *Mom* and only if he directs this communication to his Mother, not to someone else. Throughout his development, other children, relatives, and teachers will continually require increasingly refined speech from him and selectively will reinforce more and more complex sequences, until normal articulation occurs. College students who major in English or in public speaking know that intelligible expression may be the beginning for creating complex prose and words of poetry. Language begins with babbling. Many inconsistencies and errors occur in the normal acquisition of language because this process, called *Shaping* behavior, is neither deliberately planned nor consistently carried out.

Shaping also may produce undesirable activities. For example, a child's parents unintentionally may increase the intensity of his nagging (e.g., its loudness) as he continually requests some object. His mother or father may give in initially when the child's commands are moderate. Later, when he nags again, his parent may decide to behave toughly but may comply after a period of loud nagging. If appeasement happens several times, and each time the child's badgering becomes louder before he receives the reinforcer, tantrumlike behavior eventually will be shaped. In short, the parent can unwittingly develop undesirable behavior. There are many acts occurring frequently and intensely that can, in part, be explained by Shaping (e.g., bullying, cheating for more and more on one's income tax, and white-collar crime).

Thus, shaping is a powerful technique, and it can be used intentionally or unintentionally. Whenever the nurse wishes to build verbal or motor behaviors in a patient, especially in a withdrawn, nonverbal one, Shaping has applied value. If the behavior has not occurred previously, if it is no longer occurring, or if it very rarely takes place, then Shaping can be implemented.

Shaping produces a behavior by positively reinforcing an individual for each step he takes in its direction. Shaping proceeds stepwise, beginning with activities the individual is capable of performing (e.g., babbling) and ending with the behavior to be produced (e.g., the word *Mom*). Shaping a patient's behavior should be planned deliberately and should be carried out consistently to ensure effectiveness. The major ingredients of planning and implementing Shaping procedures for any patient are as follows:

Specify the Behavior to Be Shaped. The target behavior should be specified, and an analysis of its essential parts should be made. By progressively mastering each of these elements, the patient eventually can learn the target behavior. For example, suppose the long-range goal of a behavior modification program is to teach a withdrawn mental patient, who has not taken meals independently since his admission into the hospital, to eat without assistance. The first target behavior in the program, let's say, is to have the patient *walk to the dining area unassisted* by the nurses. The essential parts of this target behavior involve *taking steps (moving) in the direction of the dining area.* Suppose the dinner announcement is given over a loudspeaker located near the diningroom. If, initially, the patient turns toward the loud speaker, at this point Shaping starts. The statement by a nurse that dinner is ready also may serve as the beginning, provided that the patient turns toward the sound of the nurse's voice. *Shaping begins with a behavior the patient can perform that is in the direction of the target behavior.* That is, Shaping begins with an act that, when strengthened, increases the likelihood that the target behavior will occur (or brings the patient closer to being able to perform the target behavior). Turning toward the loudspeaker located near the diningroom involves approximating the target behavior (walking unassisted into the eating area). By mastering this first activity and all those in the direction of the target behavior, the patient will eventually be able to perform it (walk to the eating area by himself).

Find a Potent Reinforcer. Before the actual Shaping procedure can begin, however, a potent reinforcer must be found.

Administer the Reinforcer Contingent on Each Behavior That Is in the Direction of the Target Behavior. The reinforcer chosen must be administered immediately following each act (step) in the direction of the target behavior. Thus, if the patient, (in the example above) can turn toward the sound of the speaker, this movement should be reinforced without delay. As the individual begins to progress closer to the sound, each of his steps in this direction should be reinforced instantly. Gradually, he will learn to walk unassisted toward the dining area. Acquired reinforcers, such as tokens, or primary reinforcers, such as small bits of food, may be used to shape behavior.

Shape Behavior at a Moderate Speed. *Do not progress too slowly.* No act should be reinforced so many times that the patient becomes satiated with the reinforcer or that the next step becomes difficult to attain; that is, no one step should be strengthened so often that progress toward reaching the target behavior becomes slowed. Excessive reinforcement for any one step reduces the likelihood that the patient will perform the next step. Thus, when he (in the example above) hears the loudspeaker, he may turn toward it. Initially, this behavior should be reinforced. Then it becomes necessary to raise the requirement for reinforcement. Because turning behavior has been strengthened, a new behavior, such as taking a step toward the loudspeaker, very likely will occur; now this action should be required for reinforcement. Simply turning toward the loudspeaker no longer should be reinforced specifically. In other words, if only the turning behavior is strengthened, only it will occur, and the target behavior will not be reached. Consequently, the nurse continually must encourage ever increasing steps toward the final (target) behavior. *Do not progress too rapidly when shaping behavior.* If advancement is too fast, and if the demands placed on the patient are too great, the target behavior will not be reached. Thus, if after the individual has learned to take three steps toward the dining area, the nurse were to require 50 steps before she would administer the next reinforcer, the patient might even quit turning toward the sound of the speaker. Many of the behaviors already shaped would stop occurring, and the patient might give up entirely.

The nurse must know when to reinforce the particular step in the program, how many times to reinforce it—as well as when to stop reinforcing it—and to require the patient to perform the next step. Since mastering any step is predicated on becoming proficient in doing the previous one, the Shaping progression must not be too rapid or too slow. Each new action may be thought of as an extension of the previous one, and the target behavior consists of the sum of all the preceding parts. Advancing too rapidly or too slowly interferes with mastering and with extending the elements necessary for performing the target behavior. The judgment of the nurse regarding the speed of Shaping, which her previous experience aids, serves as an indispensable guide.

Once this target behavior (e.g., unassisted walking) can be performed, the other elements of independent eating can be shaped; that is, after walking into the diningroom unassisted has been shaped, sitting down at the table, properly holding utensils, placing food on them, and eating can be dealt with separately.

Various desirable complex behaviors that involve many steps can be built through Shaping. If the target behavior falls within the physical capabilities of the patient, it can be developed. The treatment definition of Shaping is as follows:

Shaping is a procedure for producing a behavior in order that the Positive Reinforcement method may be implemented for accelerating it. To accelerate the target behavior by making reinforcers contingent on it, it must occur. Shaping behavior means reinforcing the essential elements of the target behavior. The target behavior is produced by providing reinforcement for steps (actions) that move progressively closer to it.

To shape behavior effectively, it is important to understand the following: Each behavioral step must be mastered before the next, more difficult one, can occur; the target behavior should be specified before the Shaping procedure begins, and an analysis of its elements should be made; the initial behavior (the starting point of Shaping) should be delineated; the reinforcers used in strengthening each element from the beginning act to the target behavior should be potent and should be delivered immediately; progressing from the first step to the final target behavior should be neither too fast nor too slow. Shaping begins with an act the individual can perform and ends with the target behavior.

Instructing Behavior

Instruction is a part of our daily living. We read about how to assemble objects that we purchase and about how to mix accurately the ingredients of a recipe; or we listen to an individual explain how to find a street we're looking for, and so on. Instructions may be written, spoken, or given by gestures (e.g., beckoning a loved one to come forth by extending your arms). Instructions may be presented clearly (e.g., technical writers' descriptions) or confusingly (e.g., directions to an out of the way restaurant).

Nurses can use and have used instructions for many different patients with diverse health problems. For example, they effectively have employed directions for teaching patients with arthritis, with coronary conditions, with ulcers, with colostomys, or with paralysis how to care adequately for themselves. Furthermore, nurses have found instructions serviceable in helping adult psychiatric patients to learn new behaviors as well as in teaching disturbed children various activities and groups of individuals health-care practices.

For example, Putt (1970) demonstrated the usefulness of instructions in treating 36 male and female patients with peptic ulcers. The author compared the effectiveness of three nursing-care conditions: routine attention alone; routine attention plus psychological support (i.e., daily visits by the investigator with the patient, during which the professional discussed topics in a nondirective manner); and routine attention plus daily instructions concerning ulcers, their healing, and their treatment. Directions combined with routine nursing care was found the most effective of the three conditions because it reduced both the patient's discomfort and his stay in the hospital. Thus, instructions were valuable for the nurse to employ in caring for the patients. As Putt showed, the professional, nurse-practitioner must prepare herself to instruct patients in order to adequately deliver health services.

Instructions are *stimuli* that the nurse presents to the patient. These stimuli, which must be clear and explicit, detail the important actions that the patient must perform in order to be reinforced. *Instructions from the nurse, in other words, specify reinforceable behaviors for the patient.*

The nurse may use instructions for helping a patient to perform simple as well as complex behaviors. When the professional teaches the sick person about complex behaviors, such as colostomy care, each of the parts which constitute the involved actions requires delineation, instruction, and reinforcement. In other words, divide a complex behavior into its elements, and arrange them sequentially, beginning with step one; instruct each element (give directions about how to perform each behavior that is part of the target behavior); reinforce the correct performance of each explained element (encourage following instructions); proceed from one step to the next only when the patient masters the previous ones.

For example, inserting a catheter into the colostomy, adjusting the height of the irrigating bag, kneading the abdomen above and below the artificial anus, stopping peristalsis, using wax paper to line an abdominal support (Secor, 1970) are just some of the behaviors that may be directed for teaching colostomy care. The nurse may instruct each of these steps separately and may strengthen each one singly; reinforcement may be in the form of praise or feedback. After the patient has learned every element, the nurse may instruct all of them together and may reinforce the entire performance; that is, the nurse may direct and may strengthen the *total* colostomy care procedure once the patient has mastered each part. In other words, colostomy care is the target behavior composed of several essential parts (behaviors); their combination makes up the target behavior. When the nurse arranges these parts in a stepwise fashion from first to last, successfully performing each brings the patient closer than before to being able to perform the target behavior. By instructing him about how to perform each step in the direction of the target behavior and by reinforcing the patient after each successful performance, the nurse essentially has combined Instructing and Shaping procedures.

Teaching the patient about each step toward the target behavior eliminates waiting for him to perform it. The time-consuming task of Shaping a complex act, therefore, becomes easier if the nurse instructs each new step toward the target behavior. More specifically, Shaping, as indicated, involves reinforcing elements that lead to mastering the target behavior. Success with each new part, an extension of the previous one, brings the individual closer to being able to perform the goal. To shape the target behavior (e.g., unassisted walking), however, the nurse must wait for each new approximation to occur. For example, the patient must turn toward the sound from the loudspeaker if he is ever to walk to the dining area at the correct time. The nurse initially reinforces the patient's turning and then reinforces movements (steps) he makes in the direction of the dining area. But with Shaping alone, the nurse must wait for each of these behaviors to occur before strengthening them, and this process can be very long. If the patient can follow verbal instructions, however, the arduous task of Shaping may become easier. By simply instructing the patient to take a step in the correct direction and by reinforcing him when he does so, the nurse no longer needs to wait for the act to occur.

Instructions may be employed to produce a behavior in its entirety without the need to direct its separate parts or to reinforce the patient for performing each step. If a new target behavior, for example, is easy to perform, it with all of its components may be instructed. Thus, for some individuals, taking another person's temperature is an easy task that can be instructed and successfully accomplished without breaking it down into its elements. A target behavior that is complex for the particular individual and that is not easily instructed in its entirety, however, needs to be analyzed into its components, and each step must be directed and reinforced.

It is important when directing patients about behavior to realize that *instructions are most effective if the performance of the behaviors that these instructions set the occasion for are reinforced.* If the patient is not reinforced for following instructions, he may fail at the task and the likelihood that he will follow instructions given at some later time will diminish—this result will hinder his learning other tasks. Being able to follow instructions is vital.

Some profoundly disturbed adults and children do not obey even simple directions. An important first step is to accelerate their behavior, namely, following instructions. That is, *instruction following* per se, is an activity that, at times, must be strengthened. Lovaas, Berberich, Perloff and Schaeffer (1966), for example, helped disturbed children to learn new behaviors *by first teaching them to follow instructions.* Once these children could do so (once instruction following became strong), they could be taught other behaviors more easily. In short, reinforcing instruction following was the starting point for learning other activities.

Directions are helpful in caring for various patients. To use instructions effectively, however, requires more than simply providing the individual with information, as exemplified in the following treatment definition:

Describing a behavior to be performed, instructions are stimuli that the nurse gives to the patient. They should be clear, should be explicit, and should always specify exactly what behaviors are requested. Performing them should be immediately reinforced. Target behaviors easy for the patient to perform may be described in their entirety. Complex target behaviors difficult for the patient to perform should be broken down into their parts (steps) and should be arranged sequentially. Then each element should be instructed and its performance should be reinforced. Proceeding to a new step should occur when the patient has mastered the preceding ones. Once each of the steps constituting the complex behavior has been learned, all of them may be instructed, and the performance of the entire behavior may be reinforced.

The difficult task of Shaping a complex behavior may be made easier if it is possible to instruct the person to perform each of the steps that constitute the behavior.

Demonstration–Imitation

The role of imitation in human development is a fundamental one. Being able to mimic the demonstration of another, that is, being able to engage in behavior closely resembling the activity which another person has just exhibited is essential to normal development. Thus, a child's acquisition of language is partly related to his ability to mimic his parents and others. His parents shape his language, but he also learns by imitation; that is, the child observes (hears) his parents name things, imitates what he hears, and usually receives reinforcement for a correct reproduction. It is understandable that the hearing loss of deaf children prevents them from learning to imitate sounds and, therefore, often retards their speech development; early detection of this handicap is important. Children with hearing problems demonstrate crucial signs (behaviors) that trained nurses can detect (Goda, 1970).

Demonstration–Imitation, as a procedure useful in producing behavior, may be employed for many patients. With this method, in contrast to Shaping, the necessity of waiting for a particular step to occur in the direction of the target behavior becomes eliminated. One way to avoid having to wait for an activity to occur is to present instructions for it. Another way is to demonstrate it. For example, to teach a diabetic how to prepare an insulin injection, the nurse may show the procedure (may prepare the injection), and the patient may imitate it (may prepare the injection himself). The nurse should reinforce the patient's successful performance; she may employ praise and feedback valuably in this instance.

If the required target behavior is simple to learn and if the patient is cooperative, all the steps may be demonstrated at one time. If the required target behavior is complex, each of the elements must be designated, must be arranged in a stepwise fashion from first to last toward the target behavior, and must be demonstrated. And the successful imitation of each step must be reinforced. A complex behavior such as operating a dialysis machine at home may be taught in this fashion. (This machine is vital to the patient who experiences kidney failure.) Once all the steps are mastered, the entire operation may be demonstrated and its successful performance may be reinforced. Careful monitoring by the nurse in all phases of this kind of teaching is, of course, essential.

The critical features of Demonstration–Imitation are, therefore, as follows: Designate the target behavior; in a stepwise fashion beginning with the initial element, list the constituents of the target behavior; clearly demonstrate each step; reinforce the patient for each step he imitates correctly; advance from one element to the next only when the patient has mastered the previous ones. The reinforcers used in Demonstration–Imitation are determined by the patient's preferences; feedback and praise from the nurse are especially potent consequences for many patients. When all the steps involved in the complex activity can be correctly performed by the patient, the entire target behavior may be demonstrated by the nurse, and its imitation by the patient may be reinforced.

Instructions usually form part of Demonstration–Imitation. Directions such as "watch this," or more detailed ones which describe and explain the behavior to be shown usually precede each step. After observing the demonstration, the patient again may receive instructions, such as "you try it," or "do this." Furthermore, the required behavior may be described once more and the reinforcer, promised for a correct imitation, may be specified. Explicitly naming what the reinforcer will be, if the behavior is imitated correctly, is particularly useful with children or with adults who seem uncooperative.

The Demonstration–Imitation procedure is valuable for teaching vital health-care practices and may be employed usefully for teaching retarded and psychotic patients various speech and motor behaviors. Methods that utilize demonstration and imitation have been employed to reduce fears and ritualistic behaviors which trouble many individuals (see Bandura, 1969).

As indicated, the ability to imitate what others demonstrate is vital for normal development. A child's acquisition of speech is related in part to his ability to mimic the speech of others. Perhaps, those individuals without hearing problems who do not talk at all or who talk infrequently and unintelligibly may learn speech by being taught to imitate how others articulate sounds.

Several investigators have undertaken this project. Sherman (1965), for example, helped a mute adult mental patient to reacquire speech by demonstrating sounds and by reinforcing the patient for correct imitations. One difficulty Sherman encountered was that the patient at first would not imitate those exhibitions involving speech. To overcome this problem, Sherman began at a low level of imitation. More specifically, the patient's abilities were strengthened by initially teaching him to copy motor movements, such as standing and sitting, and then those involving the facial area, such as blowing and hissing. Gradually, Sherman helped the patient to extend his imitative skills to encompass oral communication, that is, to mimic speech demonstrations. Teaching a patient to talk by teaching him to imitate sounds, therefore, may have to begin by teaching him to *imitate per se*. Once he can reproduce motor behaviors (e.g., sitting), it is possible to teach him gradually to mimic sounds. The rationale is the following: If simple imitations can be produced, imitation per se (a behavior) can be reinforced. When imitation itself becomes a strong behavior, speech can be taught through imitation. The transition, however, from simple motor duplications to verbal ones, at times, is difficult (Baer, Peterson, and Sherman, 1965; Sherman, 1965). Lovaas (1967) has detailed specific steps useful for nurses involved in helping mentally disturbed children to learn to speak; his procedures rely heavily on speech-imitation teaching.

In sum, Demonstration–Imitation may be employed effectively with different patients for a variety of objectives (e.g., teaching health-care practices to the physically ill, rehabilitating the multiply handicapped, or producing verbal and motor activities in retarded as well as in psychotic patients). The appropriate use of Shaping, Instructing, and Demonstration–Imitation for producing behavior requires that the nurse be cognizant of their procedural differences. The treatment definition of Demonstration–Imitation is described as follows:

Demonstration–Imitation is one procedure that may be used in helping a patient to produce a behavior. By observing the nurse clearly demonstrate an activity and by being reinforced for correctly imitating it, a patient can learn a new behavior or can increase the complexity of some other one that he can already perform. If the activity to be produced and then to be accelerated is complex, the following steps are valuable: (1) specify the target behavior, and sequentially arrange the parts which compose it, from first to last; (2) demonstrate each part clearly; (3) reinforce the patient's correct imitation of each element shown; (4) advance from one step to the next only when the patient masters the previous ones. When all the parts can be performed correctly, they may be linked together to form the whole target behavior, which is then demonstrated in its entirety. The imitation of the total target behavior becomes the requirement for reinforcement (e.g., for setting up and for operating the dialysis machine unassisted or for saying an entire word after each of its separate sounds have been demonstrated, imitated, and reinforced).

Instructions may be used to facilitate Demonstration–Imitation. With complex behaviors, the combination of Instructing and Demonstration–Imitation reduces the tediousness resulting from completely relying on Shaping to produce the target behavior.

Guiding and Fading (Implementing and Removing Behavior Supports)

Guiding and *Fading* are two techniques that may be usefully combined to produce a behavior in individuals who either have difficulty performing the activity or simply cannot do it, even if it is carefully demonstrated or instructed. Guides are used in numerous situations. For example, some crippled patients are helped to walk by first providing them with physical supports (e.g., crutches); some profoundly retarded children are kept alive by spoon feeding them (this act is also a crutch); some patients are taught to speak through initially guiding their imitations of simple motor behaviors. In short, Guiding is useful for different purposes with different patients. The goal, however, is to help the individual to produce the desirable behavior, himself. Guiding is only a temporary step.

There are several ways to guide behavior. *Guiding may involve physically steering the patient through the behavior.* Thus, if a child is instructed, "tap the table" and is unable to follow this request, his hand may be tapped on the table. This guide would be manual. *A verbal guide would also, in a sense, steer the patient through the behavior.* Thus, if an adult is told the answer to a question he is asked, this information is a guide to producing the answer. More specifically, suppose you ask "What is this?" while you hold up a complex part of a computer. A strong verbal guide would be first to tell the adult the answer. Then eventually he, unassisted by the verbal guide, will be able to repeat the desired response. This practice is frequently used in education.

Guiding behavior whether manually, verbally, or by some other method functions as a temporary step for producing behavior. The procedure for eliminating guides is called Fading. *Fading-out refers to the gradual removal of behavioral guides.* Once they are gone, other stimuli must come to occasion the behavior. For example, if you ask the question, "What's this?" when you show an adult a complex computer part, eventually you want him to be able to answer without any help, that is, without the assistance of the verbal guide (telling him the desired response). The goal is for the question "What's this?" and for the sight of the part to set the occasion for the answer. To reiterate, the guide controls the occurrence of the behavior—it forces the behavior to occur. To transfer the control over the activity from the guide to the stimuli that you want to set the occasion for the behavior (instruction or demonstration), you must fade-out the guide and must add these other stimuli.

It also is possible to *gradually* institute stimuli that come to set the occasion for behavior—*Fading-in.* For example, a parent can be taught to assume progressively more responsibility for treating his own offspring. At first, a professional therapist, functioning as the principal behavior-change agent, may interact with the child in specific ways. Later, the parent can begin to assume some of the therapist's functions and, gradually, can take over as the principal behavior-change agent for the child. That is, the therapist's influence can be faded-out while the parent's influence is faded-in. (The importance of teaching parents to manage the behavior problems of their children will be discussed later.)

Sherman (1965) used Guiding and Fading procedures to reinstate the speech of a mental patient with problems like the ones of the person mentioned in the last section. After many hours, the patient could say "food" when shown a piece of food and when given the verbal guide, "Say food." But when Sherman originally held up the food and asked, "What is this?" the patient could not give the correct answer. To get the patient to answer the question "What is this?" without the verbal guide "Say food," the following procedure, as described by the author, was employed:

> To obtain the word "food" from the subject when the experimenter asked, "What is this?" a fading procedure was used. With the fading procedure, the experimenter continued to hold up a bit of food each time and to deliver instructions to the subject. The behavior of the subject—that is, saying "Food"—was maintained with reinforcement while the instructions to the subject were gradually changed in the following steps: (a) "Say food"; (b) "Say foo____"; (c) "Say f____"; (d) "What is this? Say f____"; (e) "What is this? Say ______"; (f) "What is this?"[11]

---

[11]J. A. Sherman, "Use of reinforcement and imitation to reinstate verbal behavior in mute psychotics," *Journal of Abnormal Psychology*, 70, 1965, 158.

After many sessions, the patient could say "food" as soon as it was shown and as soon as the appropriate question was asked. Thus, by beginning with a verbal guide that urged the occurrence of the behavior and then by gradually Fading-out this instruction and by introducing the question "What is this?" the patient eventually learned to answer correctly. This procedure involves more than simply being able to imitate speech.

Guiding and Fading may be employed to produce a behavior if the following principles are followed: Tell the patient what you want him to do (e.g., "Touch my hand") and tell him what reinforcer will be given if he follows the instruction (e.g., "I'll give you a sip of coke"); guide the patient through the behavior (e.g., lift his hand and touch it to yours; immediately reinforce the patient; repeat this sequence several times and fade-out the manual guidance (e.g., gradually lessen your hold on the patient's hand as you touch it to yours) until the instruction alone leads to the behavior. Precisely how fast this guidance is faded-out depends on the patient. Enough steering must be used each time, however, to make the behavior (e.g., touching your hand) occur.

To illustrate once again the Guiding and Fading procedures, another example (Berkowitz, Sherry, and Davis, 1971),[12] which concerns teaching self-feeding to profoundly retarded children, will be presented. Spoon-feeding retarded children is a laborious activity. Also, it is certainly not in their best interests to spoon-feed them when they can be taught to become more independent. The aides in this study were shown how to steer each youngster's self-feeding behavior as well as how to fade-out these guides. The reinforcers used in this study were praise, "pats on the back," and food. Successful completion of each step was followed by reinforcement. Apparently the stimuli that gradually occasioned self-feeding were (1) being served the meal and (2) having eating utensils available. The self-feeding procedure was described as follows:

1. Aide, holding child's hand with spoon in child's hand, makes entire feeding cycle, from plate (scooping food) to mouth and back to plate.
2. Aide makes entire feeding cycle, but partially releases child's hand (still holding spoon with food on it) 2–3 inches below child's mouth. Child lifts spoon these last few inches himself.

---

[12]Samuel Berkowitz, Patrick Sherry, and Barbara Alphin Davis, "Teaching self-feeding skills to profound retardates using reinforcement and fading procedures," *Behavior Therapy*, 2, 1971, 62–67.

3. Aide releases child's hand approximately six inches from child's mouth. Child lifts spoon about six inches.
4. Aide scoops food, releases child's hand at plate level. Child lifts spoon from plate to mouth.
5. Aide brings child's hand to plate, releasing hand. Child scoops food, and lifts spoon to mouth.
6. Aide releases hand after child has emptied spoon. Child brings spoon down to plate, scoops food, and lifts to mouth.
7. Child executes entire self-feeding cycle by himself.

> On the 1st day of the training program, the aide stood behind the child, holding the spoon tightly in his hand and feeding him as he sat facing the plate of food on the table (step 1). This procedure was followed for all three meals of this 1st day. On the first meal of the 2nd day, after repeating the above procedure several times, the aide introduced the first variation (step 2) in the fading procedure. Now the aide let go of the child's hand about 2–3 inches from the child's mouth. The child was now required to move the spoon these few inches to get his reinforcement.
>
> Upon the successful completion of step 2 for at least one entire meal, the aide advanced to step 3, terminating her grip and movement at a distance still further from the child's mouth and closer to the plate of food, thus requiring the child to lift the spoon a greater distance. With each step, the child succeeded in performing more of the self-feeding cycle by himself and required less assistance from the aide. The aim was to ensure success by making the steps small and by not trying to advance the child too quickly.[13]

The results were successful. The authors concluded that if a child can hold a spoon and can lift it from his plate to his mouth, he may be taught to feed himself.

Guiding and Fading procedures may be incorporated into programs for helping patients to learn many motor as well as verbal activities (e.g., self-care behavior, speech). Guiding and Fading are also applicable in physical therapy. The nurse may employ these procedures for assisting the disabled patient in adjusting to the recent onset of a physical handicap. That is, the nurse may use Guiding and Fading to reduce the sudden despair and futility that a newly handicapped individual feels by helping him to acquire competence in an activity with which he is having difficulty (e.g., writing with his left hand after his right arm has been amputated).

---

[13]Ibid., pp. 64–65.

This behavior may be taught by manually Guiding the patient's left hand, by gradually Fading-out the manual assistance (e.g., by gradually lessening your grip on the patient's hand), and by praising or by giving him feedback for each of his successes. The patient progressively will acquire the ability to perform the behavior himself, unassisted by the nurse.

Fading, in this situation as in all others, should occur gradually so that stress for the patient is minimized. The speed of Fading the guide depends on the patient's progress, not on the nurse's wishes. The treatment definitions of Guiding and Fading are as follows:

Guiding and Fading are procedures used to produce behavior. Guiding refers to either physically or verbally steering the individual through the behavior, and Fading refers to eliminating this support. Control over the behavior may be transferred from the guide to other stimuli (instructions or demonstrations) by Fading-out the guide. The steps involved in Guiding and Fading are these: First, present the desired stimulus (e.g., an instruction to the patient concerning the desired behavior); second, provide a support for the behavior (e.g., manual or verbal guide); third, reinforce each occurrence of the desired behavior; fourth, repeat these steps and fade-out the support until the desired stimulus alone leads to the behavior. Provided that the transition from the support to the desired stimulus—the guide to instruction—is gradual, the stress for the patient will be kept at a minimum (very few failures will occur). The speed at which the guide is faded-out or a new stimulus is faded-in depends on the progress of the patient.

Linking

Human beings behave in complex ways. A person can perform several activities in close succession, if the entire series is necessary for a positive reinforcer to be administered. To change a person's conduct in desirable ways, however, behavior modification purposely segments complex sequences into simpler units—into single acts. The best way to help a patient is to understand his separate behaviors. Although human activities must be simplified—must be divided into manageable units—the behavior modification approach does not deny or does not overlook complex sequences of behavior; quite the reverse is true.

Through principles, such as chaining, an attempt to understand complex sequences of behavior can be carried out. A chain is a series of behaviors that ultimately leads to reinforcement. Each separate activity in the chain is related to the one preceding it and to the one following it. For example, consider the description which one dialysis patient gave:

> For three years Kenneth Stewart's early-morning routine, every Monday and Thursday, has been the same—arrive at the Manhattan Veterans Administration Hospital dialysis unit, hurriedly change in the locker room, weigh himself, take his temperature, record the results, and be ready for nurse Audrey Foy to take his blood pressure.[14]

Changing in the locker room, weighing in, taking his own temperature, and recording the results are all behaviors that this dialysis patient performs two mornings each week. To understand this sequence, we need to know what events set the occasion for and strengthen each behavior in the chain. The most potent reinforcers occur at the end of the series—dialysis treatment and, in turn, remaining alive. The most apparent stimuli which begin the series of behaviors—which set the occasion for it—are the particular days of the week, Monday and Thursday. In short, on Mondays and Thursdays, this patient drives to the hospital, changes his clothes in the locker room, and so on; that is, he engages in a chain of behaviors in order to receive dialysis treatment and, thereby, to stay alive.

Each activity in the chain produces a stimulus that has two functions. First, it acts as a reinforcer for this behavior—the behavior that produced it. Second, it sets the occasion for the next activity in the series. More specifically, each behavior in the chain leads to the production of a stimulus that reinforces this behavior and, at the same time, that sets the occasion for the next one. For example, consider driving to the hospital. This activity is reinforced because it results in the patient's arrival at the institution. He drives there to get there—driving to the hospital produces the stimulus, being at the hospital. In addition, being at the hospital sets the occasion for the next behavior, changing clothes in the locker room. This behavior results in being undressed—a stimulus—which reinforces the activity of changing clothes. Also, this stimulus sets the occasion for weighing (the next behavior in this chain). The chain may be analyzed into even smaller units, but the logic would remain the same.

Consider another example, namely, reciting Longfellow's "Prelude to Evangeline." The verse flows smoothly from the individual

---

[14]"Two days of every week," *American Journal of Nursing,* 70, No. 1, 1970, 77.

who, while alone, recites it from memory. Each word is reinforced by the sound it produces for the speaker; and, in addition, each word sets the occasion for (triggers) the next one in the series. This flow of words would be markedly disrupted if the speaker tried to recite the poem backward. Since each word does not set the occasion for the previous word, reciting the poem backward would be difficult, at least initially. The major points of the discussion are these: *Series (chains) of behavior occur regularly; each behavior in the chain is reinforced by stimuli it produces; these stimuli set the occasion for the next behavior in the sequence.*

For behavior modification, the notion that activities can be linked together is a useful one. All behavior modification procedures involving Shaping attempt to produce a chain of behaviors. Thus, the different ones associated with dining independently, (e.g., walking into the dining room unassisted, sitting down at the table) must eventually be connected. The entire process of eating self-reliantly after hearing the call to dinner may be thought of as a complex chain of behaviors. Also, the *result* of teaching a person to operate a difficult machine (e.g., Instructing his behavior, reinforcing his performance of each step and combining them into one unified performance) is a chain.

Developing a complex sequence of behaviors after each one in the sequence has been strengthened separately is desirable. What follows is a description of how a sequence of behaviors can be taught. (This description, however, is not a technical analysis of the process termed *chaining*.)

It is possible to join two or more behaviors after each has been strengthened separately, that is, it is possible to link behaviors together. For example, each morning a mildly retarded child may be instructed to get ready for breakfast. The child may be taught that, after this instruction is given, if he brushes his teeth, he will earn one token; teeth brushing can be produced and can be accelerated through Positive Reinforcement. The token may be used as payment for some preferred activity. A second behavior, bed making, may also be accelerated through receipt of a token, if the child makes his bed after he is told to do so. Thus, both of these activities may be instructed individually, and their occurrences may be reinforced separately; both activities may be strengthened apart from each other.

One valuable extension of this self-care program is to *link* together these two behaviors—teeth brushing, and bedmaking—both may be required before the reinforcer (one token) would be administered. More specifically, the child may be instructed to get ready for breakfast. After this instruction, he would have to brush his teeth and to make his bed in order to receive the token.

If this program were carried out, the two behaviors would be linked together so that the opportunity to make the bed and, thereby, to receive one token would be available only if the child brushed his teeth. Cooperation would be followed by the opportunity to make the bed, resulting in his receiving a token. The two activities would be connected because both would be necessary for the reinforcer to be administered. In fact, only if the first one were performed *correctly* would the opportunity to perform the second one be given; that is, only if the child brushed his teeth satisfactorily would he be allowed to make his bed and, thereby, to receive a token. Thus, greater complexity can be introduced by *Linking* behaviors together. The treatment definition of this procedure is as follows:

Linking together behaviors means joining two or more in a sequence wherein the last activity is followed by a potent reinforcer. Each activity is strengthened separately through the Positive Reinforcement procedure. Then, the behaviors are joined together two at a time such that the opportunity to perform the second one and, thereby, to receive the reinforcer becomes contingent on correctly performing the first one. The occurrence of each is followed by the opportunity to perform the next one. The last behavior in the series is followed by the potent reinforcer.

Two activities, each separately strengthened initially, may be joined together in this fashion. Once the sequence occurs regularly, a third behavior may be added. Thus, a child may have to brush his teeth, to make his bed, and to dress himself before extrinsic reinforcers would be administered. The complexity of an individual's activities can be increased in this manner. Sequences of behavior can be produced and can be accelerated.

In sum, this part has considered five approaches for *producing* behaviors so that they can be *accelerated*. The applications which follow illustrate these methods:

Application 5. Using Shaping to Help a Mental Patient to Regain His Speech

The patient in this study (Isaacs, Thomas and Goldiamond, 1960)[15] was a very withdrawn and inactive 40-year-old man who had been in a mental hospital for 19 years (he would sit almost motionless where he was situated). After being placed in the hospital, he

---

[15]Wayne Isaacs, James Thomas, and Israel Goldiamond, "Application of operant conditioning to reinstate verbal behavior in psychotics," *Journal of Speech and Hearing Disorders*, 25, 1960, 8–12.

became mute and remained this way during the entire 19-year period. No physical reason why this patient had lost his ability to speak was apparent. To accelerate speaking, this behavior first had to be produced. Consequently, Shaping procedures were employed. Briefly, the authors developed the patient's speech by reinforcing his facial movements. To illustrate the Shaping procedure, the author's methods are presented below. (In this discussion the letter *S* refers to the patient and the letter *E* refers to the experimenter. Also, the term *successive approximation* means Shaping.) As the authors described:

> The *S* was brought to a group-therapy session with other chronic schizophrenics (who were verbal), but he sat in the position in which he was placed and continued the withdrawal behaviors which characterized him. He remained impassive and stared ahead even when cigarettes, which other members accepted, were offered to him and were waved before his face. At one session, when *E* removed cigarettes from his pocket, a package of chewing gum accidentally fell out. The *S*'s eyes moved toward the gum and then returned to their usual position. This response was chosen by *E* as one with which he would start to work, using the method of successive approximation. . . .
>
> The *S* met individually with *E* three times a week. Group sessions also continued. The following sequence of procedures was introduced in the private sessions. Although the weeks are numbered consecutively, they did not follow at regular intervals since other duties kept *E* from seeing *S* every week.
>
> Weeks 1, 2. A stick of gum was held before *S*'s face, and *E* waited until *S*'s eyes moved toward it. When this response occurred, *E* as a consequence gave him the gum. By the end of the second week, response probability in the presence of the gum was increased to such an extent that *S*'s eyes moved toward the gum as soon as it was held up.
>
> Weeks 3, 4. The *E* now held the gum before *S*, waiting until he noticed movement in *S*'s lips before giving it to him. Toward the end of the first session of the third week, a lip movement spontaneously occurred, which *E* promptly reinforced. By the end of this week, both lip movement and eye movement occurred when the gum was held up. The *E* then withheld giving *S* the gum until *S* spontaneously made a vocalization, at which time *E* gave *S* the gum. By the end of this week, holding up the gum readily occasioned eye movement toward it, lip movement, and a vocalization resembling a croak.

> Weeks 5, 6. The *E* held up the gum, and said, "Say *gum, gum,*" repeating these words each time *S* vocalized. Giving *S* the gum was made contingent upon vocalizations increasingly approximating *gum.* At the sixth session (at the end of Week 6), when *E* said, "Say *gum, gum,*" *S* suddenly said, "Gum, please." This response was accompanied by reinstatement of other responses of this class, that is, *S* answered questions regarding his name and age.[16]

Thus, Shaping was successful in producing speech. Shaping began with a behavior the patient could perform (e.g., moving his eyes toward the gum) and ended with his performing the target behavior (e.g., speech). Each step between these two activities had to be reinforced positively enough so that it could serve as the basis for the next step. Thus, eye movements preceded lip movements, and lip movements preceded vocalizations (croak). The croak preceded speech (the word, *gum*). Each step had to occur before it could be reinforced, and each step was an extension of the previous one. The potent reinforcers were administered promptly, and Shaping was neither too fast nor too slow.

According to the authors, once the statement, "Gum please," occurred, other verbal behaviors also began to take place. For example, the patient would respond to questions about his name and age. This process is generalization, that is, other speech in addition to the statements specifically accelerated began to occur. This generalization also was accompanied by generalization to other people (people other than the experimenter) and to other situations (situations other than where treatment took place); the patient began to talk to nurses and to others with whom he was involved in various places. To increase markedly the frequency of this individual's speaking, however, he would have to be consistently reinforced when he spoke and consistently not reinforced when he did not speak. The authors noted that the patient did not speak to individuals who interpreted his nonspeech behaviors, who did not require him to talk.

Other examples of Shaping procedures can be found. Rice, McDaniel, and Denney (1968) used Shaping procedures for a six-year-old retarded child with severe cerebral palsy; arm movements were reinforced with spoonfuls of ice cream. The value of Shaping in producing both motor and verbal behaviors for severely withdrawn and for nonverbal patients cannot be overemphasized. As indicated,

---

[16]Ibid., p. 9.

other behavior-producing procedures (e.g., Instructing behavior) may be combined with Shaping; where applicable, a combination is advantageous.

Application 6. Instructing and Reinforcing Smiling in a Retarded Child

Smiling is a simple activity that a person is likely to engage in when he encounters another person. Smiling may occur in various situations, but generally it is directed at another individual; therefore, it is a social behavior. When we notice that another person rarely smiles in social situations, we may conclude that he is rude or unfriendly. When we observe lack of smiling in a retarded or mental patient, however, we usually consider it a manifestation of his problem. The judgment, which frequently occurs, that deficient social behavior is a sign of a patient's problems is one important reason for its elimination.

A lack of social behavior in retarded children contributes to society's setting apart. It seems valuable, therefore, for the nurse to accelerate their social behaviors so that the differences between them and other children become attenuated. In addition, adequate social skills are necessary for capably living in society. The child in this example (Hopkins, 1968)[17] was eight-years old and retarded; he attended a class for retarded children in a research school at a university. As described by the author, when the child encountered other people he would not smile but instead would remain "straight faced."

Treatment took place in the outside environment of the school wherein the author, the child, and an observer took walks. Each walk continued until ten different people who greeted the boy were encountered. Treatment lasted for 76 days. The procedures used to *produce* smiling, then to *accelerate* it, and finally to make it *durable* are presented below:

PRELIMINARY PROCEDURES. During the first five walks, an attempt was made to find out how often the child smiled when he met another person. Since it was found that he never smiled, the Positive Reinforcement procedure was instituted; that is, for the next five walks, the child was immediately given a piece of candy if he smiled at a person who greeted him. Again, it was found that the child

---

[17]B.L. Hopkins, "Effects of candy and social reinforcement, instructions, and reinforcement schedule leaning on the modification and maintenance of smiling," *Journal of Applied Behavior Analysis*, 1, 1968, 121–129.

never smiled. This result was predictable. *If the behavior never occurs, how can it be accelerated?* To strengthen smiling by administering positive reinforcers (e.g., candy), it was first necessary to produce the smiling behavior.

A time-out procedure was also implemented during this period —that is, if the child failed to smile, the person he was walking with would turn away from him for a few seconds. This punishment is used to decelerate undesirable behavior, in this case, not smiling. (See Chapter 4, Section 4.2).

PRODUCING AND THEN ACCELERATING SMILING. To produce smiling each time the child encountered anyone, he was instructed, "Smile, when you say hello to ______." The use of instructions during these nine walks led to increased smiling. But this effect did not last for very long; that is, instructions were effective only in producing the behavior initially. To increase the frequency of smiling once it had been developed required reinstitution of the Positive Reinforcement procedure. For the next 21 walks, therefore, each time the child smiled at an individual who greeted him, he was given a piece of candy, which resulted in increased smiling. In other words, the *Positive Reinforcement procedure was ineffective at the beginning of the study because the behavior never had occurred; and, therefore, it could not be reinforced. After instructions were used to produce the behavior, however, Positive Reinforcement was successfully reapplied.* Notice that the effectiveness of Instructing smiling was directly related to the consequences of smiling; that is, this activity was positively reinforced.

ASCERTAINING IF CANDY CAN BE REMOVED WITHOUT THE SMILING BEHAVIOR DECREASING. The child cannot be reinforced with candy for the rest of his life each time he smiles. Eventually, the reinforcer must be abandoned. From the forty-first through the forty-sixth walk, therefore, using sweets was completely discontinued, which unfortunately resulted in a rapid decrease of smiling. Perhaps, the transition from continuous candy reinforcement to no such reinforcement was too abrupt. As will be indicated in Section 3.5, a behavior strengthened on a continuous schedule—each occurrence of the behavior is followed by administration of the reinforcer—is unlikely to remain strong if the administration of positive consequences is stopped *suddenly*. But, if it is discontinued *gradually*—tapered off—the activity is more likely to remain strong once the reinforcer is discontinued completely.

GRADUALLY STOPPING THE ADMINISTRATION OF THE CANDY REINFORCER. To recapture the behavior, candy was re-introduced as the reinforcer for smiling during the next nine walks. After the behavior had once again become strong, the administration of candy was gradually stopped. More and more smiling had to occur before the reinforcer was administered; that is, the reinforcer was given after five or after seven smiling behaviors, for instance, instead of after each one. Progressively increased smiling was required before a reinforcer was delivered. Now, when the candy was stopped completely, the behavior did not decrease as it had done previously.

Two additional conditions were employed in this study to test whether social reinforcers—responses of other people to the child when he smiled—were effective in maintaining the strength of the behavior after candy reinforcement had stopped. It was found that social reinforcers were functioning in this manner. Perhaps, by gradually discontinuing the administration of candy, the author helped to bring smiling under the influence of more natural reinforcers; that is, control over the smiling may have been transferred from candy to attention from others. Social reinforcers are important in making the results of behavior modification programs durable (see Section 3.5).

In sum, Instructing the behavior of smiling was an effective procedure for *producing* it in a retarded child, but the Positive Reinforcement method was necessary to *increase its frequency.* In addition, it was found that when positive reinforcers were discontinued completely, the smiling rapidly decreased. When Positive Reinforcement was reinstituted on a continuous basis, the behavior again became strong. And when the transition from continuous reinforcement to none was made gradual, the smiling behavior *remained* strong. The author of the study concluded that *gradually* stopping the administration of reinforcers, in contrast to *suddenly* stopping them, *might* have resulted in the smiling behavior coming under the control of social reinforcers.

Application 7. Teaching Severely Retarded Girls about Grooming

This application (Treffry et al., 1970)[18] illustrates the techniques used to teach several severely retarded girls to wash and dry

[18]D. Treffry, G.L. Martin, G. Samels, and C. Watson, "Operant conditioning of grooming behavior in severely retarded girls," *Mental Retardation*, 8, No. 4, 1970, 29–33.

their hands and faces. The girls were 10–20-years old and had been living in an institution for the retarded from 1–13 years; intelligence quotients ranged from 20 to 30, which placed all the girls within the profoundly retarded range. None of them in this program had severe physical defects involving the upper extremities; so, they were physically capable of performing the washing behavior. Also, all of them were taken off medications, with the exception of anticonvulsive drugs. To produce grooming behaviors in these girls, Instructing, Guiding and Fading, as well as Linking procedures were used. In addition, two methods for decelerating undesirable behavior were employed. The target behavior for each child was successfully washing and drying her hands and face without physical guidance from the nurse. To accomplish this goal, the target behavior was broken down into the following elements:

1. Pointing to the hot water tap on command;
2. Pointing to the cold water tap on command;
3. Placing the plug in the sink;
4. Placing water in the sink;
5. Wetting hands with facecloth;
6. Washing hands with facecloth and soap;
7. Wetting face with facecloth;
8. Washing face with facecloth and soap;
9. Rinsing soap from hands;
10. Rinsing soap from face;
11. Drying hands;
12. Drying face.

The teaching sessions took place in one of the washrooms at the institution, which contained several sinks, mirrors, toilets, a cupboard for towels, and a bench for the girls to sit on. Psychiatric nurses and nurses' aides, previously instructed in basic behavior modification procedures, were the teachers. Before the actual instruction began, however, the patients were tested to see if they could perform the target behavior. It was found that virtually none of them could execute it in its entirety. This type of initial evaluation forms a necessary part of a well designed behavior modification program; it will be discussed further in Chapter 5. The grooming program then began. A typical teaching session is presented below. (The letters *S* and *E* stand for the retarded girl and for the experimenter, respectively. Also, the term *verbal prompt* means an instruction.)

> During any one session, from five to fifteen minutes would be spent teaching the *S* step 1 with candy and social reinforcement given for each correct response. At the end of that time, the *S* would be guided through the rest of the steps and would receive an additional candy following the completion of washing. This pattern was continued during subsequent sessions until the *S* had mastered step 1. Following such mastery, each session consisted of having the *S* perform step 1 for candy, receive training on step 2 for five to fifteen minutes, and then be guided through the remainder of the steps. When step 2 had been mastered, the *S* performed steps 1 and 2 for a candy, was trained on step 3 for a brief time and was then guided through the remainder of the steps. This pattern continued until the *S* could perform the entire grooming sequence within a session, for which she received a single reinforcer.[19]

Thus, a typical teaching session incorporated Guiding, Fading, and Linking (i.e., the entire grooming sequence was performed before reinforcers were administered; each step was linked to the next step). The target behavior, therefore, was shaped progressively by teaching the girls to perform each part unassisted. During the beginning stages, it was necessary for one staff member to teach only one pupil at a time. But, as progress was made, the individual staff members could begin working with two or three girls at a time. From a practical standpoint, this result is important.

During a teaching session, each girl was given instructions about a particular step and was guided through it. (Instructing and Guiding were combined.) After several repetitions, physical guidance was gradually eliminated (was faded-out) until instructions alone could occasion the step. Although not utilized, demonstrations in conjunction with instructions, could have been employed in this teaching; that is, each girl could have observed the staff member perform the step, in addition to her simply hearing the instruction. As previously indicated, the behavior-producing techniques of Instructing and Demonstration–Imitation can be effectively combined. The following text, which illustrates how the girls were taught to identify the hot water tap, provides a more detailed explanation:

> The staff stood the *S* directly in front of the sink and said, "Show me the hot water tap (which was painted red on top)". If the *S* held her hand on the tap with no resistance to *E*'s guidance,

---

[19]Ibid., pp. 30–31.

> she was given a small piece of candy and a great deal of social approval. Inappropriate responses to verbal prompts—or offering resistance to physical guidance were followed by a sharp "no", and fifteen second time-out (the *S* was completely ignored for fifteen seconds), following which the procedure was resumed. Certain behaviors during the time-out, such as throwing soap or abusing other children, were followed by a sharp slap on the fingers.
>
> Over a number of trials, the pressure of *E*'s hand was gradually lessened (faded-out) until eventually the *S* responded to *E*'s question, "Show me the hot water tap," by touching the tap. Following ten correct responses to the verbal prompt, *E* moved on to step 2.[20]

By employing aversive stimulation (e.g., saying no or giving a sharp slap) and time-out procedures, the nurses were able to reduce undesirable behaviors that could have prevented the girls from developing more beneficial ones. The rationale for using punishment is presented in Chapter 4. In general, both steps 2 and 3 were taught in the same way. Steps 4 through 12, however, had to be subdivided further, as exemplified below for step 4:

> Steps 4–12 had to be broken down into smaller components for effective teaching. Step 4, placing water in the sink, consisted of: turning on the hot water tap; turning off the hot water tap; turning on the cold water tap; turning off the cold water tap. Each of these responses were taught individually. . . .[21]

The remaining steps (5–12) were also segmented further into smaller units. The results of the procedures were favorable, indicating that grooming behaviors can be taught to even severely retarded patients, indeed, that they should be taught to these patients.

The suitability of behavior modification methods for accelerating desired activities in patients is evident. For the retarded, especially, these techniques have been used for toilet training, for academic skills, for self-help, and for health-care. An interesting example (Abramson and Wunderlich, 1970), which shows the application of behavior modification principles to producing and to accelerating dental hygiene practices (e.g., teeth brushing) in markedly retarded boys has been reported. The target behavior, properly brushing

---

[20]Ibid., p. 31.

[21]Ibid., p. 31.

teeth, is a complex task. To teach this behavior, the investigators employed three stages: The first focused on discrimination learning in order to teach each child to use his own toothbrush, and the second incorporated Shaping and Positive Reinforcement to produce and to strengthen certain preparatory behaviors necessary in brushing teeth. The third used Demonstration-Imitation in conjunction with Instructing and Shaping to produce correct brushing behavior. In this stage, each child was instructed first about an important element in the program, and if he performed it, he was reinforced with a token. If he could not perform the behavior, however, the Demonstration–Imitation procedure was employed; that is, the teacher demonstrated the step and, when necessary, carefully guided the child through it. Correct imitations were reinforced with praise and with tokens. The results of this hygiene program were successful; the children learned to brush their teeth.

The possible combinations of the procedures for producing behavior and their various applications are too numerous to mention here. Their potential range of usefulness by the nurse still is undetermined.

TERMS AND QUESTIONS

Terms

Shaping
Instructing
Demonstration–Imitation
Guiding
Fading-out
Fading-in
Linking

Questions

1. How are positive reinforcers used in producing behavior?
2. How would you use the Shaping procedure to produce smiling in the retarded child discussed in Application 6?
3. How would you use the Demonstration–Imitation procedure to produce smiling in this child?
4. How will you design a behavior modification program to teach a patient to eat unassisted? Let us say the patient is a 30-year-old

adult hospitalized for seven years, who, in the past, has been spoon-fed.

5. How will you design a behavior modification program valuable in the total treatment for a child with cerebral palsy?

3.5 *BENEFICIALLY IMPLEMENTING POSITIVE REINFORCEMENT: FACILITATING MEANINGFULNESS AND FOSTERING PREVENTION BY TAPERING OFF REINFORCEMENT AND BY USING SOCIAL REINFORCERS*

In this chapter, we have been concerned with procedures for producing and for accelerating desirable behavior. Undoubtedly, when the modification procedures are used appropriately, many different patients with many different problems can be helped. The Positive Reinforcement procedure is *effective* in accelerating behavior, which means that large changes result (Baer, Wolf and Risley, 1968). The modified activity is *relevant* if most individuals in society would judge it important (see Chapter 1). Effectiveness and relevance are two important requirements of behavior modification programs and, for that matter, of any approach to patient care. Another equally important requisite is *meaningfulness.* A behavior modification program is meaningful to the extent that the following take place:

The Desirable Changes in Behavior Accomplished in One Situation Also Occur in Others. For example, if a mentally retarded patient is helped to learn routine hygienic practices, such as bathing himself and brushing his teeth, during his stay in the institution, these daily self-care behaviors must continue when he moves to a new situation, such as the home. In addition, if a mental patient can carry on relevant and coherent conversations with the nurse instrumental in strengthening this activity, he must continue to carry on logical conversations with other individuals, such as relatives, physicians, and other nurses. Thus, other people must be able to occasion desirable behavior from the patient in addition to the specific nurses involved in his treatment. The extent to which the results of a behavior modification program *generalize* (see Section 3.1) to new situations and to other people is one measure of meaningfulness.

The Breadth of Behavior Change Is Extensive. This statement means that other desirable behaviors begin to occur, in addition to the ones specifically accelerated. For example, suppose Fading and

Guiding have been employed successfully to help a recently handicapped patient to use his left arm for writing. If other behaviors (e.g., drawing) begin to occur without the nurse applying behavior modification procedures to them, generalization has occurred. The extent of it—the number of related activities strengthened without specifically being reinforced—is an indicator of meaningfulness.

THE RESULTANT CHANGES ARE DURABLE. Changes in behavior that continue after the behavior modification program has ended are lasting ones. If a nurse is successful in helping a patient to behave more capably than before by accelerating his desirable activities, the question concerning durability of change becomes crucial. Short-lived positive results are only demonstrations of effectiveness—the positive results of treatment should last. Without durable behavior change, the occurrence of either type of generalization mentioned above becomes unlikely. Thus, if the retarded patient's hygenic activities do not persist, they cannot occur in new situations; and if the behavior of the handicapped patient, which entails using his left arm, does not last, the occurrence of other (new) activities, which also require the use of the patient's left arm, will be improbable. In short, the generalization of the accelerated behavior to new situations, and its generalization to new behaviors will be unlikely if the positive effects of behavior modification do not last. (Patterson, Ray, and Shaw, 1968). With permanent outcomes, however, both these other circumstances become more probable; that is, generalization to new situations and to new behaviors is, to some extent, predicated on durable results.

THE ACCELERATED BEHAVIORS ARE USEFUL FOR THE PATIENT IN HIS INTERACTIONS WITH HIS ENVIRONMENT. Many patients, notably those in mental hospitals, lack behaviors essential to living capably in the outside community. Budgeting money, purchasing clothing and nutritious food, developing friendships, and various other self-directed activities that involve decision making exemplify behaviors which should become the focus of a behavior modification program *at some point* during a patient's stay in the hospital. To help him behave more capably than before requires that activities necessary to his existing *in the outside community* be strengthened, not just those essential to running the ward smoothly. Self-directed decision making eventually must replace the usual subordinate role of a mental patient, which means that the nurse has to reduce her influence over the patient's behavior and has to help him to make important decisions himself. This attempt at meaningfulness will be discussed in Chapter 7, and in the Concluding Statement. The importance of contacting existing sources of positive reinforcement in the natural environment will be discussed in Section 3.6.

THE PATIENT LEARNS SELF-CONTROL. This aspect of meaningfulness resembles the previous one. Self-control, a relevant topic for treating many patients with varying problems, involves specific procedures that the nurse may employ for helping an individual to learn how to change and to control his own behavior—he can become his own therapist (Goldiamond, 1965). Teaching a patient self-control (see Concluding Statement) will result in *durable* effects with respect to the behavior being treated, in *broad* effects with respect to preparing the patient for handling other problems that are troubling him, and in *preventative* effects with respect to stopping the unbridled occurrences of new problems.

The following reflect meaningful behavior modification: behavior changes that occur in several situations; behavior changes that generalize to activities other than the ones specifically accelerated; behavior changes that are durable and persistent; behavior changes that are useful for the patient in his interactions with the natural environment; behavior changes that help the patient to gain self-control. The remainder of this part and all of Section 3.6 is concerned with these issues, particularly with the ones pertaining to durability and to generalization of behavior changes. Preventative alterations, which center around the nurse as a teacher, will be an important aspect of this discussion. What follows is an examination of two techniques that facilitate durability and generalization. These may be incorporated into a behavior modification program.

Reinforcing the Target Behavior Intermittently (Tapering)

In Section 3.3, it was stated that neither too much nor too little reinforcement should be used in a behavior modification program. Furthermore, it was recommended that the quantity of reinforcement be plentiful in the early stages but that it then be reduced gradually. Thus, if ten tokens initially are given to a patient, after he has performed the target behavior, the number of tokens contingent on the behavior should be reduced gradually; eventually, only one token has to be used. This strategy will help to avoid the problems of the therapist running out of reinforcers and of the reinforcer losing its potency. In addition, it is likely that reducing the amount of reinforcement used in this manner will result in the behavior remaining strong once it has been accelerated, even though reinforcement is at a minimum.

Another way to accomplish reduction is to decrease the number of times the reinforcer is administered, that is, to taper off reinforcement. Recall that when each occurrence of the behavior is followed by the reinforcer, the schedule is continuous (see Section 3.3). As indicated, a continuous reinforcement schedule is the most efficient one for accelerating a behavior. Intermittent schedules (schedules in which reinforcement is not continuous), however, are the most effective ones for making behavior persist after reinforcement is discontinued completely—the behavior no longer produces the reinforcer. With intermittent schedules, in contrast to continuous ones, reinforcers are *not* administered after each occurrence of the target behavior. Two intermittent schedules are discussed below:

THE VARIABLE RATIO SCHEDULE. With this schedule, reinforcers are administered after a number of behaviors greater than one have occurred. For example, suppose a nurse wants to help a somewhat withdrawn mental patient to talk more frequently with the other patients. Initially, to increase the frequency of this behavior, the nurse reinforces the individual (e.g., administers tokens) *each* time he is seen conversing with the other ward members. This schedule is a continuous one in which reinforcers are administered 100% of the time. When the behavior becomes strong, the nurse administers reinforcers less frequently, perhaps after nine out of ten such activities. More specifically, the nurse provides reinforcers after 90% of the occurrences of the target behavior—90% of the time. This procedure is a variable ratio reinforcement schedule. The nurse gradually may increase its intermittence by administering reinforcers, on the average, for five out of ten occurrences of the target behavior. If this plan were implemented, reinforcement would result, on the average, 50% of the time, that is, after half the occurrences of the target behavior. The frequency of reinforcement may be decreased; that is, reinforcers may be administered, on the average, about 33% of the time—a reinforcer would follow one out of three occurrences of the target behavior. Administering reinforcers may be made extremely intermittent, such as one for every 100 occurrences of a particular activity.

Thus, the variable ratio schedule involves not having reinforcers follow each occurrence, but rather some average amount of behavior. The term *ratio* means that some *amount of behavior* greater than one activity must take place before the reinforcer is delivered. The term *variable* means that, *on the average*, the reinforcer is delivered for the amount of behavior (ratio) designated; that is, the ratio is not followed strictly. For example, if the variable ratio schedule includes five behaviors for one reinforcer (Variable Ratio 5), on the average, five activities must occur before the one reinforcer is administered. *Notice, however, that when the reinforcer is administered it follows one of the behaviors.* Even if the variable ratio schedule were extremely intermittent, and, on the average, only one in one hundred of the behaviors were followed by the reinforcer, still, when the reinforcer was delivered, it immediately would follow the occurrence of one of the behaviors. Remember, reinforcers should always be contingent on behavior and for best results should be administered immediately after an activity occurs.

THE VARIABLE INTERVAL SCHEDULE. This schedule focuses on the amount of *time* passing between reinforcements. Thus, the patient described above may have been given a reinforcer following his talking with the other patients if, let us say, ten minutes had elapsed *since his last talking behavior was followed by a reinforcer.* Twenty or 30 talking behaviors may have occurred during this ten-minute interval. But the only talking behavior followed by the reinforcer would have been the one occurring soonest after the end of this period. Again, it is important to notice that the reinforcer follows the behavior; the reinforcer is not just given at the end of ten minutes per se. *The reinforcer is given following the target behavior which occurs soonest after the end of the ten-minute interval.*

Interval, therefore, means time between reinforcements. Variable, in this example, means that, *on the average,* ten minutes must pass between the administration of reinforcers. Thus, sometimes nine minutes go by, and sometimes eleven minutes elapse. But on the average, the first behavior that occurs after ten minutes of no reinforcement is followed by the reinforcer. (The designated time between reinforcements is not strictly obeyed.) Variable interval schedules may be mildly, moderately, or extremely intermittent. An extremely intermittent variable interval schedule is one in which a long period (e.g., two hours), on the average, elapses between the delivery of reinforcers, even though there may be many occurrences of the target behavior.

Several reasons may be given for why the nurse should strive to make the administration of reinforcers *progressively* more intermittent.[22] First, the behavior modification program becomes *eco-*

---

[22]This discussion of simple intermittent schedules is concerned only with variable schedules. Fixed schedules (e.g., fixed ratio—wherein a *consistent* number of occurrences of the behavior greater than one is required before the reinforcer is administered—

nomical (Reese, 1966). The more intermittent the schedule of reinforcement (either variable ratio or variable interval), the fewer the reinforcers used. Very intermittent schedules, therefore, are very economical—only a few reinforcers are administered for many behaviors; the nurse is unlikely to run out of reinforcers. Second, the behavior modification program is *less likely to be hampered by satiation* with respect to the reinforcer. They will retain their potency longer if only a few are administered, which is especially true for primary reinforcers.

Third, as indicated, the target behavior will *continue to occur longer* after the reinforcers used to accelerate it have been discontinued completely. More specifically, if during the behavior modification program, the schedule is gradually made more intermittent, the target behavior will persist longer, once the reinforcers used to accelerate it are removed, than if only a continuous schedule has preceded this discontinuation of reinforcement.

If reinforcers are delivered on variable schedules, a person does not know when to expect them, and he will continue to perform the behavior steadily; that is, the administration of reinforcers, from the patient's point of view, is not predictable; in such a situation, he is likely to continually perform the behavior. For example, if a child nags his mother for candy and the mother only *occasionally* gives in, the nagging behavior will occur very often. Let us suppose that the mother gives the child candy, on the average, once every fifty times he asks for it. The effect of intermittent reinforcement on the nagging behavior will be to perpetuate it at a high frequency; that is, when the child wants candy, he will repeatedly ask for it. Speaking nontechnically, we may say he knows he will get candy if he asks for it, but he does not know exactly how many times he must demand it. This arrangement is a variable ratio schedule of reinforcement. Mother may also accelerate her child's nagging by using a variable interval schedule. For instance, Mother may give in, on the average, once every thirty minutes. She may give her child candy following his demands about every half hour. In either case, the results would be the same: steady nagging. In general, the effect of administering reinforcers on variable schedules is to cause the behavior to occur steadily without interruption. And when the reinforcers used to accelerate the behavior are removed completely, it will continue to occur for a long period of time.

All things being equal, any activity will tend to occur longer

---

and fixed interval—wherein a *constant* period intervenes between the administration of reinforcers), however, are also intermittent schedules. For a thorough explanation of fixed schedules, see Ferster and Perrott, *Behavior Principles*, 1968.

once the reinforcer used to accelerate it is removed, if the administration of reinforcers has previously been intermittent rather than just continuous. For example, a quarter slot machine pays off intermittently. On the average, for every 100 quarters you insert, let us say, the machine hits the jackpot once (variable ratio schedule). Sometimes 500 quarters are put into the machine, and sometimes 20 quarters are enough for the jackpot. Observation of participants will show that, very often, they will play one machine for hours. Occasional reinforcements (pay offs) prolong the activity and keep it at a high frequency. Thus, the slot machine player continues for a long time, despite infrequent reinforcement. If the machine breaks down (if it gives no more jackpots), he will probably continue for hours before eventually giving it up entirely. On the other hand, if for some reason a particular slot machine always returns money on every play (a very profitable schedule) and then *suddenly* ceased, the individual will be likely to soon stop playing it. If reinforcement is discontinued completely after an intermittent schedule has been in effect, the behavior will continue to occur for a longer period than if previously only a continuous schedule had been used. Intermittent schedules produce more durable behavior than continuous ones.

As will be discussed in the next section, many desirable activities can be prolonged for *extended* periods if they can come under the control of *social reinforcers* such as praise and attention from others. Tapering off the administration of reinforcers such as candy or trinkets, which (in conjunction with social consequences) have been presented contingent on some target behavior, may be a vital step in a behavior modification program that, in part, is aimed at converting praise and attention from others into effective reinforcers (see Application 6; Allen and Harris, 1966; and Wahler, 1968).

In sum, the administration of reinforcers contingent on behavior during some portion of the modification program should be made more intermittent (either by a variable ratio or by a variable interval schedule). The reduction in the overall number of reinforcers administered—this process is called *tapering* or thinning—must be gradual. If the reinforcers are decreased gradually, the desired behavior will occur regularly for fewer and fewer reinforcers, and the patient will be less likely to grow tired of them. And when the reinforcers initially used to accelerate the behavior are completely discontinued, it will be more likely to remain frequent than if no tapering had previously taken place.

To accelerate behavior, reinforce it continuously. To help to make it durable, reinforce it intermittently. The strategy to use, therefore, is this one: *initially follow each occurrence of the behav-*

ior with a reinforcer; then, after the behavior is taking place frequently, make the administration of these reinforcers gradually more intermittent. If the nurse proceeds too fast in making the reinforcement intermittent, however, the behavior may decelerate. (Relatedly, if the nurse starts with a schedule in which the reinforcers are administered too infrequently, the behavior may never become accelerated.) Guides as to how gradually the nurse should make reinforcement progressively more infrequent are difficult to state. The most preferable approach is to keep a close check on the behavior. If it starts to diminish in frequency, perhaps reinforcement is too sparse. In this case, the nurse should back up and should present more frequent reinforcement. The judgment of the nurse and the records of the patient's behavior (see Chapter 5) are helpful in this situation as well as all other aspects of behavior modification.

Substituting Social Reinforcers for Material Reinforcers

Primary reinforcers (e.g., food) or other material ones (e.g., trinkets) should eventually be eliminated from the treatment program, and social reinforcers (e.g., praise and attention), found in the natural environment, should be substituted. Social reinforcers are naturally occurring reinforcers; that is, people in the natural environment use them. Consequently, how durable will be the results of the behavior modification program will be influenced by how potent these reinforcers become for the patient—that is, how responsive he is to social consequences. In the natural environment, social reinforcers usually follow the patient's desirable behavior, not reinforcers such as those imposed arbitrarily in a behavior modification program. Furthermore, social reinforcers are likely to be withdrawn if the person misbehaves or is deficient in his behavior. Therefore, they must become powerful consequences for him. If he is unresponsive to them, he will be unable to live capably in the community.

Social reinforcers play a major role in both the desirable and undesirable behaviors of many people. In children, for example, these reinforcers have been found to perpetuate both objectionable (Harris et al., 1964) and pleasing behavior (see Application 6). The difference involves contingency; that is, social reinforcers following undesirable behavior (e.g., a tantrum) can perpetuate it in the same way that social reinforcers can maintain desirable behavior. Using social reinforcement appropriately, therefore, is vital.

As mentioned previously, many patients are unresponsive to praise and to attention from others. For these individuals, notably psychotic children and extremely withdrawn adults in mental hospitals, social consequences, such as being with others or being praised for an accomplishment, are rarely reinforcing. Accelerating desirable behavior requires the nurse to first implement primary (e.g., food) or material reinforcers (e.g., trinkets), because social stimuli (e.g., praise and attention) do not function as reinforcers. Social events, however, can gradually be made into reinforcers; indeed, this goal should be one for the treatment of a socially unresponsive patient. Lovaas, Freitag, Kinder, Rubenstein, Schaeffer, and Simmons (1966) have reported a procedure for establishing social reinforcers in schizophrenic children; the most important part involves making social events the occasions for the delivery of food. The youngsters were extremely disturbed and unresponsive to social stimulation, such as being told "good." All nurses caring for autistic children should read about the complex methods that the investigators developed for converting social consequences into reinforcers.

For many individuals, if praise from the nurse is coupled with administering primary reinforcers, praise can be transformed into a potent reinforcer, as indicated in Section 3.2. For clarification, suppose the target behavior for working with a particular disturbed nonverbal child, is designated as naming objects correctly. To convert approval into a potent reinforcer, each correct activity the child performs should first be commended and then should be followed immediately by a primary reinforcer (e.g., food). As the behavior becomes strengthened, *the food gradually should be eliminated from treatment*, whereas praise from the nurse should continue to follow each correct activity. With this procedure, social approval alone is likely to become a potent reinforcer. Since most people are not praised *excessively* each time they do something positive, the approval given to the patient should not be overdone so that it becomes dull or phony (see Section 3.3); moderation is especially important once the patient becomes responsive to social reinforcers. In the initial stages of behavior modification, more than one nurse and more than one treatment setting should be employed to broaden (to generalize) the influence of social reinforcers; the patient has to be able to respond to different people in different situations in order to develop various socially relevant behaviors.

Responsiveness to social reinforcers is essential for capable functioning with other people; therefore, developing the strength of these reinforcers may be useful in perpetuating a positive change in the patient's behavior. For example, the positive effects of behavior modification proved durable when a five-year-old girl, whose body was covered with open sores and scabs resulting from scratching, was helped with the Positive Reinforcement procedure (Allen et al., 1966), which incorporated both trinkets and social approval as positive consequences. In the beginning of this program, the child's mother was told to reinforce her daughter with praise and with trinkets contingent on desirable nonscratching behaviors (see Reinforcing Incompatible Behavior in Chapter 4). Thus, behaviors not involving scratching were to be accelerated. As the scabs and the sores began to heal and to disappear, the mother was told to gradually eliminate the trinkets as reinforcers—reinforcement became increasingly intermittent. Social approval, however, still followed each time she did not scratch herself; that is, social approval was kept continuous. Gold stars were also given to the child for desirable behavior; they were retained in the program as reminders for the mother to pay attention to her child's desirable activities. The meaningfulness of these procedures, particularly the use of social reinforcers, was revealed by a four month follow-up report showing that the scars and scabs remained absent.

In sum, social reinforcement is important to use for all patients. For those unresponsive to praise or to attention from others, one objective of the behavior modification program should be to convert these consequences into potent reinforcers. Social reinforcers not only can help to make the positive results of behavior modification durable but also can increase the likelihood that other desirable activities will occur in other appropriate contexts. By coupling social consequences with reinforcers that already are potent, the nurse can make social consequences into reinforcers that will be able to accelerate desirable behaviors. This principle is useful for numerous behavior problems a nurse may encounter in the natural environment, such as helping a family (LeBow, 1972), as well as working in the hospital setting. Increasing the potency of social reinforcers is but one step toward assisting many patients in achieving improved adjustment.

TERMS AND QUESTIONS

Terms

Meaningfulness
Durability
Tapering off reinforcement
Intermittent schedule
Variable ratio schedule
Variable interval schedule

Economy (in a behavior modification program)
Social reinforcer

Questions

1. Gambling (e.g., playing slot machines) is a behavior reinforced on a variable ratio schedule. On what type of schedule is the following activity reinforced: looking down the street for your friend while you are waiting on a corner for him to pick you up and to drive you to school? Explain.
2. An intermittent schedule was used in Application 6 (increasing smiling) to make behavior more durable. Was this schedule variable interval or variable ratio? How do you know?
3. How may a patient's complaining about aches and pains be accelerated inadvertently on a variable interval or on a variable ratio schedule? Discuss.
4. Why should social reinforcers be used for patients?
5. How can you teach a ten-year-old child to respond to your approval? Explain. Assume that, initially, the child generally does not respond to this consequence.

3.6 *BENEFICIALLY IMPLEMENTING POSITIVE REINFORCEMENT: FACILITATING MEANINGFULNESS AND FOSTERNG PREVENTION BY UTILIZING OTHER HELPING AGENTS AND SOURCES OF BEHAVIOR MODIFICATION*

Behavior modification is a flexible approach that may be useful for teaching health-care behaviors to patients with physical illnesses and for ameliorating the condition of individuals with behavior problems. In this part, four ways involving behavior modification principles in the origination of durable and generalized changes as well as in the prevention of undesirable activities will be proposed.

Using Behavior Modification Principles to Teach Individuals, Families, and Large Groups Health-Care Behaviors

Efforts toward perpetuating and extending the positive effects of any treatment that a patient receives in the hospital helps to make that treatment meaningful. One essential responsibility of the nurse is to foster continuation and extension of results. This responsibility, in part, can be met by health teaching. Educating a patient's family as well as the patient about how to continue and to extend treatment procedures in the home may be vital. For example, a wife may need instruction about the appropriate foods to cook for her husband, who is receiving treatment for a peptic ulcer. Or parents may need instructions concerning the necessary procedures for dealing with their cerebral-palsied child; the nurse may need to demonstrate how braces or night splints, or orthepedic shoes are put on the child. Or parents may want to know how they may assuage the feelings of brothers and sisters who feel neglected when most attention is paid to the sick child.

Whatever the specific problems, the procedures advised must be put into *concrete behavioral terms*; they must not be left as vague assertions. Thus, instead of telling a mother that the brothers and sisters of the sick child should be loved more, the nurse should list specific behaviors that these siblings may perform in order to feel included. She should describe the reinforcers, contingent on these activities, that the mother can administer. Generally, all the behaviors which the nurse considers appropriate for the parents to perform may be *instructed, demonstrated, and shaped,* and must be *reinforced contingently.*

Both the patient and his family can be taught the crucial health-care behaviors necessary for his recuperation. Basically, a family-centered approach involves teaching the members of the family what helpful, concrete behaviors they must perform.

For example, parents not only can be taught what exercises their crippled child must perform but also how they can "motivate" and can encourage him to perform these health-care behaviors. Translated, parents can learn to use potent reinforcers effectively.

By educating parents about how to care for their sick child or a husband about how to care for his ill wife or vice-versa, the nurse will be instrumental in perpetuating and in extending the progress made in the hospital. Effective teaching results from using some basic behavior modification principles—namely, Instructing, Demonstration–Imitation, Shaping, Linking, defining goals as target behaviors, analyzing their elements (if necessary), applying reinforcers on a contingent basis, and so on—that is, when the behavior modification approach is employed, the desired behaviors of specific family members necessary for the recuperation of the sick member can be strengthened. Parents or a spouse may become the principal treatment agent for the sick member of the family.

The cooperation of the family members in correctly performing certain activities must be reinforced (praise and feedback) by the nurse. Precise monitoring of their progress also is required (see Chapter 5). Therefore, the parents or the spouse may need to learn to keep records of his treatment activities so that the nurse can administer reinforcers for successful performances. When a child is the patient, accurate monitoring and immediate reinforcement can be accomplished if the nurse observes the parents' interactions with the child at home. By observing the mother, for example, help the crippled child with his exercises or put on his orthepedic shoes, the nurse can give both corrective feedback or further demonstrations as well as praise for accurately carrying out the designated activities.

In addition, the patient may be taught to become the principal treatment agent for himself. Many individuals can be taught to continue to care for themselves and to maintain their own health. Thus, a diabetic can learn to administer his own injections or a physically disabled person can learn about his dietary needs and about the essential exercises he must perform at home. Likewise, someone recovering from a radical mastectomy can learn exercises she can perform at home. Teaching is useful during a patient's stay in the hospital and when he returns home. If he learns to care for himself, the positive gains made in the hospital will be more likely to become durable. Reinforcement for the patient's performance of the health-care behaviors he is taught usually derives from his success with the behaviors he attempts and from his knowing that he is caring for himself effectively. For some patients, however, this type of reinforcement is not enough, and specific procedures must be employed to help the patient to help himself (see Concluding Statement). Patient teaching is a dynamic process that nurses in the hospital setting as well as in the community environment must perform (Aiken, 1970; Aradine and Hansen, 1970).

For many years health teaching and nursing demonstrations for the patient and for his family have occurred primarily in the home. Home visits, however, not only are costly, they also may be unrealistic, particularly in view of the limited number of highly prepared professional nurse-practitioners existing in relation to the large number of individuals requiring health education. The question confronting nurses who work in the community is whether a way exists for reaching many people with the limited number of qualified nurses available. One possibility involves teaching (Remillet and Reading, 1970) groups of individuals with similar chronic illnesses (e.g., diabetes) who can learn about self-care. Another related possibility deals with teaching groups of nonprofessionals (e.g., home health aides) who live in the community and who can and want to participate in caring for patients. As Remillet and Reading propose, these assistants can be educated in helping the nurse-practitioner with the delivery of home health services. A health-aide may be an important member of a nursing team in a neighborhood health center, for instance, not only because of the help he or she provides to nurses teaching health care in the home or in the clinic but also because of the knowledge he or she has about the language, the life styles, and the areas of sensitivity in the community (Shannon, 1970). In either case (teaching groups of people with similar chronic illnesses or groups of people who can be mobilized as assistants), the nurse extends the range of her services. With more people being reached, more benefits will accrue.

Teaching in the community also may result in steps taken toward prevention and toward early detection of various illnesses. That is, by educating residents about health practices involving sanitation and nutrition or by teaching them to recognize impending signs of illnesses, such as glaucoma and diabetes, the nurse can foster prevention and early treatment. Similarly, by educating parent groups about detecting and treating child behavior problems, the nurse can help make prevention from omnipresent difficulties, such as juvenile delinquency, more feasible.

Therefore, teaching is a crucial function of nursing in the *hospital* (e.g., preoperative and postoperative teaching); in the *schools* (e.g., teaching health-care practices and developing curricula concerned with instruction); in the *homes*; and in the *community* at large. No matter what specific behaviors are being taught, or who is being taught (e.g., the individual patient, the family, a group of individuals with the same chronic illness, community residents interested in improving the health practices in their environment, or group of health-aides), effective and meaningful teaching is essential.

To accomplish this goal, the Positive Reinforcement procedure and the techniques for producing behavior can be usefully applied. Some general guides for teaching health-care behaviors follow. These guides are garnered from the information contained in this text. *First,* the behaviors to be taught must be defined as *target behaviors. Second,* the students should be *instructed* in every behavior. If these activities are complex, each of their elements should be instructed. Practice in performance should be reinforced, and errors should be corrected. Demonstration–Imitation can be employed effectively in combination with Instructing behaviors. Demonstration–Imitation coupled with a careful utilization of feedback and praise produces a very effective teaching package. Complex activities divided into their parts can be eventually chained together. In short, the techniques for producing behavior can be profitably used for teaching health-care practices. *Third,* the nurse should *monitor all activities.* Families, patients, and health aides can be taught the importance of keeping precise charts of the various specified procedures, or the nurse can *directly observe* these treatment agents performing the necessary activities during a home visit. With both approaches, the nurse can monitor progress and can correct errors. *Fourth,* the cooperation and the increased skill of the treatment agents always should be reinforced.

To facilitate the teaching process with groups of people, the instructor should assign readings about the behaviors being taught. These passages should be accompanied by *study questions* constructed in order to illuminate the more important aspects. After each group member has read the material and has answered the study questions, the members may form pairs and may discuss the material with each other. Then a group discussion would be valuable. Talking about the material in these ways gives the nurses and the group members themselves an opportunity to recognize and to remedy any misunderstandings or other problems. These suggestions are based on research indicating that behavior modification principles can facilitate the teaching process (see Ferster and Perrott, 1968).

Behavior modification principles may be used not only for teaching participants about health care practices but also for maintaining the participation of individuals at these group meetings. Many will continue to attend gatherings because of the information and knowledge they expect to acquire. For them, the transmission of information about health-care behaviors, part of the long-range goal of the group, acts as a potent reinforcer. For other people, frequently those in poverty areas, knowledge and information about health-care practices may not initially be potent enough reinforcers to maintain attendance; thus, at important group meetings, it may be low in the beginning stages. Strengthening attendance, therefore, may be an essential first step for the nurse involved with organizing a productive health-teaching group.

In this regard, a study by Miller and Miller (1970)[23] is pertinent. To strengthen attendance of welfare recipients at self-help group meetings, these authors employed supplementary reinforcers, such as "used furniture," "finding jobs for teenagers," and various

---

[23]L. K. Miller and O. L. Miller, "Reinforcing self-help group activities of welfare recipients," *Journal of Applied Behavior Analysis,* 3, 1970, 57–64. Copyright 1970 by the Society for the Experimental Analysis of Behavior, Inc.

types of information. By defining attendance at self-help group meetings as the target behavior and by making the administration of supplementary reinforcers contingent on it, Miller and Miller could maintain the participation of poverty-stricken individuals. As the authors stated:

> These supplementary reinforcers allowed for the systematic scheduling of meaningful consequences that would maintain individual participation until other naturally available reinforcers can develop control. Such supplementary reinforcers may be imperative during the initial phases of an organization when it is not yet strong enough to guarantee group success.[24]

The use of supplementary reinforcers for group attendance may be necessary for teaching residents of deprived areas about nutrition, prenatal care, venereal disease, drug abuse, hygiene, and other important health topics. Tokens given for attending meetings and redeemed for various other reinforcers also could be employed productively. The main point is that attendance and participation in group gatherings may initially need to be defined as target behaviors and strengthened by the Positive Reinforcement procedure in order for other events, such as receipt of knowledge about health care behaviors, to eventually become potent reinforcers.

Teaching Behavior Modification Principles to Other Helping Agents (e.g., Parents, Schoolteachers, and Foster Grandparents)

For a patient with behavior problems, the likelihood that the positive effects of a behavior modification program will be durable and will generalize after it terminates is related to the type of environment he encounters. More specifically, if after the behavior modification program has ended, the patient is placed in an environment where reinforcers are made contingent on his desirable behaviors, it is likely that these activities, which were accelerated in treatment, will last and will occur in situations other than the one where they were accelerated. In addition, it is probable that other desirable behaviors will begin to take place. The environment of the patient directly influences his behavior.

There are several environments in which children and adoles-

---

[24]Ibid., p. 63.

cents spend much of their time. Two of the more important of these are the home and the school. What follows is a discussion of the need for educating significant members of the child's and adolescent's environment—other helping agents, such as parents and teachers—to reinforce desirable behavior contingently, which will result in these individuals becoming better reinforcement agents—administrators of reinforcement—for children and adolescents. Desirable adult behavior similarly may be the focus of any discussion having to do with altering the reinforcement practices of the environment and with teaching behavior modification, but since the majority of research involves child and adolescent behavior problems, the following discussion will concern these age groups.

The family environment can contribute to both the prosocial and the deviant behavior of children and adolescents. Helping the child or the adolescent with behavior problems not only may involve specific attempts to modify his or her behavior *per se,* but also may involve attempts to *alter the reinforcement practices of the family environment.* For example, Conger (1970) was able to alter the reinforcement practices of a mother in relation to her nine-year-old son and, thereby, was able to reduce the child's behavior problems. He was soiling himself from one to four times a day. Since examinations had revealed no medical problem and since dietary changes had no effect on his soiling behavior, the mother was told to stop paying attention to the problem; that is, the mother was told to "no longer wash and change" the boy "or to give attention via verbal interchange." The child was told to take care of himself if and when he dirtied himself. This procedure was employed because it was believed that the child's behavior was being reinforced by the mother's attention; that is, the mother would react sympathetically and would wash and change the child after he had dirtied himself. Therefore, the mother was told to discontinue attention previously contingent on soiling behavior (see Extinction, Chapter 4), and instead was told to make attention contingent on nonsoiling behavior. This switch in contingencies or rearrangement of social reinforcers reduced the problem to zero.

Thus, instead of treating the child's behavior problem per se, the mother's responses to the problem were altered. This change in the reinforcement practices durably reduced the undesirable behavior. Although the mother in this example did not grasp fully the rationale involved in the behavior modification program, the procedures, nevertheless, were effective. In short, the activities of children and adolescents are modifiable by changing parents' reinforcement practices. Conger's treatment for the child mentioned above was centered in the environment where the behavior problem was reinforced; altering reinforcement practices proved to be a productive strategy.

A related strategy, which also seeks to alter the reinforcement practices of the family environment but which, in addition, provides parents with the rationale involved in the behavior modification program, entails teaching parents behavior modification per se. Parents, in other words, learn to produce, to accelerate, to maintain, and to extend the occurrences of desirable behavior as well as to prevent severe relapses and other behavior problems from arising. Mental-health care practices, therefore, can be instructed. Teaching mental-health care behaviors to families involves *teaching parents how to formulate their own behavior modification programs and how to extend ones already being implemented for their children.*

Teaching parents how to manage the activities of their children is useful not only for dealing with current problems (e.g., aggressiveness, withdrawal) but also for dealing with future ones. Although current difficulties can be changed by Instructing the parents to alter their present reinforcement practices, as illustrated by Conger's example, future problems or relapses into "old" ones can be prevented from getting out of hand *if the parents are taught to implement new procedures or to reinstitute previously effective ones.* If productive behavior modification practices (e.g., paying attention to desirable behavior, not to undesirable behavior) are incorporated into the daily child-rearing activities of parents and also into the educational activities of school teachers, many appropriate behaviors can be developed and inappropriate ones prevented. *Relapses,* for example, can be dealt with by reinstituting previously successful procedures (see Application 1). It is reasonable that relapses in previously modified behaviors can occur; that is, unwanted social behaviors can be revived, and desired social behavior can be reduced after treatment ends, if a breakdown in the reinforcement practices of parents occurs. Thus, if after the unpleasant crying of a child has been reduced, although not completely eliminated, a parent runs into the child's room when the child cries—the parent mistakenly administers positive reinforcers—the behavior will reappear in full force (e.g., Williams, 1959). Similarly, if a child is reinforced for interacting with his mother and this social behavior becomes more frequent (previously this interaction between mother and child had rarely taken place), the mother's momentary preoccupation with other activities may cause a reduction in the social behavior. In either case, a parent with knowledge of behavior modification principles can re-apply previously successful procedures, which will make the relapse only temporary.

Furthermore, if new problems begin to develop, or if new desirable behaviors are wanted, a parent with knowledge of behavior modification principles can implement specific procedures for achieving the desired goals. Thus, parents with a retarded child living at home can be instrumental in teaching him many wanted activities, such as feeding himself, bathing, toileting, counting money, and ways of beginning to interact effectively with his peers. All these and others can be accelerated by the judicious use of the Positive Reinforcement procedure. No matter what the age of the child (i.e., whether he is a preschooler or of high school age) teaching his parents practices of altering behavior is valuable as a step toward preventing the unbridled occurrence of problems and as a way to make behavior modification meaningful.

Other advantages of educating parents include both a reduction in the nurse's time spent supervising behavior modification programs and, relatedly, an extension of her influence over other families with difficulties. Thus, if parents are taught behavior modification principles, they can carry out the program for their child without the continuous supervision of the nurse being necessary. Parents taught appropriate methods for managing and for improving the behavior of their children can become effective treatment agents for long periods, which increases the likelihood of durable and general behavior changes occurring. Also, since supervision by the nurse may become less frequent for any individual family, the range of usefulness of the nurse in helping other such groups to deal with their problems becomes extended. In other words, by helping parents to alter their reinforcement practices, which may be maintaining undesirable activities, and by teaching mothers and fathers about behavior modification principles per se, the potential of parents as effective reinforcement agents becomes increased. And for children and adolescents with behavior problems—whether frequently occurring undesirable ones, such as being overly aggressive, or deficits in behavior, such as found with the retarded–educating parents may be crucial. The nurse can help children and adolescents meaningfully by teaching their mothers and their fathers, who can help them continually, about behavior modification practices so that they will become improved reinforcing agents. This method is a *family-centered approach.*

Not only parents but also different family members, school teachers, peers, and others can be enlisted in a total-environment approach (Patterson, McNeal, Hawkins, and Phelps, 1967). The school, in particular, is extremely fertile both for modifying and for preventing behavior problems, notably juvenile delinquency. Since a relationship exists between early difficulties in school and later juvenile delinquency (Fredlund, 1970), it is logical that the nurse responsible for bettering the health of school children should involve herself in helping to prevent their misbehavior. Fredlund has listed several ways in which the school nurse may participate in the prevention of delinquency. Among these are working with parents, children, and teachers, as well as developing curricula in the school. Providing education for parents and helping to develop courses having to do with family living and child growth, which incorporate the teaching of behavior modification principles, are pertinent to the nurse's role in preventing delinquency and other problems. As Fredlund points out, direct action must be taken if anything is to be done about juvenile delinquency. Educating others about behavior modification principles pertains to the role of the nurse both in remedying existing social problems and in preventing future ones.

Teaching foster grandparents (LeRoux and Arlton, 1969) behavior modification is another way for the nurse to remedy many problems. Foster grandparents may function as surrogate mothers and fathers to institutionalized children. If the charge nurse in a medical setting, for example, were to mobilize the potential of elderly people for improving the condition of institutionalized youngsters by instructing the former about the basic behavior modification principles pertinent to child care, the mutual benefit to the old and young alike would be extensive.

Teaching may be accomplished individually or in groups and may take place in the home, the school, the hospital, or in various other community facilities. Regardless of how many people learn the behavior modification principles at the same time or where their education is carried out, the successful use of these tenets is more likely if the helping agents learn how to observe behavior accurately, how to record behavior precisely, and how to implement skillfully basic procedures in the best interests of the child or adolescent. Several ways of teaching behavior modification are possible. What follows are some general guides.

In essence, helping agents (e.g., parents and foster grandparents) must learn three activities. These are the target behaviors of the program.

Teach the Individual to Observe. To improve the behaviors of anyone, it is necessary to observe the following: the frequency of his activities; the consequences of his activities (what generally follows them); the events that precede his activities (the stimuli that set the occasion for them); the potential reinforcers (what activities or material objects does the person seem to like which may be effective in accelerating new desirable behavior?). The crucial events that occur before and after the activities of the child or adolescent may be produced by other persons in his environment.

TEACH THE INDIVIDUAL TO RECORD WHAT IS OBSERVED. To make use of observations, the individual must record them precisely. In Chapter 5, techniques for making exact observations and records of behavior will be discussed.

TEACH THE INDIVIDUAL TO IMPLEMENT BEHAVIOR MODIFICATION PROCEDURES. This activity involves teaching much of the information already presented in this book concerning the Positive Reinforcement procedure.

1. Behavior is strong or weak because of its consequences (its effects on the environment); that is, the frequency of a given activity, how many times it occurs in a specific situation, is related to what follows that activity.
2. Behavior also is related to its antecedents; that is, events which precede the reinforced activity can come to set the occasion for that activity. Thus, the importance of specific situations and people involved in treatment must be stressed.
3. Reinforcers should be contingent on behavior; that is, the performance of the target behavior should result in the reinforcer.
4. Several kinds of reinforcers—events that strengthen the behavior they follow—may be used. Primary reinforcers (e.g., food), acquired reinforcers, generalized-acquired reinforcers (e.g., praise and attention), and activity reinforcers may be employed in a behavior modification program.
5. Reinforcers should be potent.
6. Reinforcers should be administered immediately.
7. Neither too much nor too little reinforcement should follow the behavior.
8. The administration of reinforcers should be on a continuous schedule to accelerate behavior (each occurrence of the behavior should be reinforced).
9. Reinforcers should be administered sincerely.
10. For many institutionalized children, a period of adaptation to the treatment situation and to the change agent (e.g., foster grandparent) may be necessary.

After the Positive Reinforcement procedure has been explained, it is advisable to teach the helping agents how to employ some of the basic methods useful in *producing* and in increasing the complexity of behavior (e.g., Shaping, and Linking). Techniques for making changes durable and general (see Section 3.5) should also be taught. Furthermore, where appropriate, the use of the Negative Reinforcement procedure may be explained (see Section 3.7). Finally, the helping agents may be taught how to employ some of the deceleration techniques (e.g., time-out, extinction). They are useful for reducing frequently occurring and interfering undesirable behavior. This reduction may facilitate the acceleration of desirable behavior. Teaching individuals how to combine Positive Reinforcement with one or more of the deceleration methods is advantageous (see Chapter 4).

The three target behaviors should be strengthened sequentially from observing and recording activities to implementing procedures. The nurse may teach each target behavior. This educational process will be aided, if basic behavioral procedures useful in producing and accelerating behavior are employed (e.g., Instructing, or Demonstration–Imitation). For example, instructions may be given about how to observe some specifically defined target behavior, such as the number of times child *A* walks to within three feet of child *B*. (This information will be useful in a program for increasing the interaction of child *A* with other children.) The nurse then may show the recording procedures, and the helping agent may attempt to duplicate her demonstration. In addition, the nurse may show more difficult activities, such as administering positive reinforcers for child *A*'s interactions and approaches to child *B* (e.g., child *A* walks to within three feet and then eventually interacts with child *B*). The helping agent may then attempt to administer positive reinforcers contingent on child *A*'s interacting with child *B*. Fading also may be used; that is, the nurse gradually may reduce her amount of participation in treatment and may allow the helping agent to gradually participate more.

Conferences at the *end* of teaching sessions are important for giving both corrective feedback and reinforcement to the helping agent. During teaching, devices that signal him to strengthen a behavior or that provide him with feedback indicating that reinforcers have been administered correctly are useful (Wahler et al., 1965). In other words, behavior modification procedures may be used to teach other individuals the same methods. The three essential target behaviors mentioned above may be accelerated by the same procedures employed in accelerating other activities.

The cooperation of helping agents is vital and, if lacking, will need specific development by making the consequences of cooperation reinforcing. As stated, teaching can be accomplished in the home or in the hospital, wherein groups of helping agents can be taught at the same time. With the group approach, a wider variety of behaviors can be discussed, and more feedback about procedures and potential problems can be given. Practice in observing and in recording activities or in implementing the procedures can be assigned at home or in the hospital environment.

The teaching program can be introduced by having the helping agents read one of the programmed texts on behavior modification which are currently available (Patterson and Guillon, 1968) in order to obtain an overview of the basic principles. Once these agents are working with the children or with the adolescents, the nurse should make periodic checks for progress. This monitoring can be accomplished by analyzing the behavior charts of the change agents or, more directly, by observing them interact with the persons they are working with. Thus, behavior modification principles may be helpful in teaching other helping agents how to alter behavior.

Teaching the Patient

Aiken (1970), in a very informative article, discussed the importance of teaching the patient as an ongoing, vital process central to the hospital-staff nurse's role; the author also showed that behavior modification is useful in carrying out this process. Aiken presented two examples of instruction wherein the target behaviors, designated for each patient, were formulated on the basis of a careful assessment of both the patient's behavioral history and his current problems. In one example, a 67-year-old female in a mental hospital was treated for a malignant rectal mass that subsequently resulted in the performance of a sigmoid colostomy. Initially, postoperative teaching was considered useless because of her mental problems. After carefully assessing her *behavioral history* in the mental hospital, however, the nursing staff decided that health teaching was possible and advisable. The patient's background indicated that she was capable of performing many self-care activities (e.g., bathing, dressing). To provide her with knowledge about colostomy care, therefore, four essential parts of this behavior were accelerated. The first three: removing and reapplying a colostomy bag and cleansing the skin around the stoma, were learned quickly, which enabled the fourth step, daily regulation of her bowel with a suppository, also to be quickly accelerated. Thus, by carefully assessing this patient's behavioral history in the mental hospital, the nurses were able to formulate and teach her essential steps in caring for her artificial anus.

In another example, Aiken described the care of a 50-year-old woman hospitalized for an exploratory laparotomy for a bowel obstruction. As can be seen from the author's statements below, this patient was difficult:

> She put her light on at least every 15 minutes, day and night, for apparently unimportant reasons—she wanted her tubes checked, the drainage measured, her dressing inspected, and so on, ad infinitum. The nursing staff began to visit her less and took longer to answer her light. They avoided her, not because she caused them more work, but because they felt frustrated by their inability to satisfy her.[25]

Because they realized that this patient had previously encountered bad experiences in hospitals, and because they recognized that she was nervous and upset about the possibility of complications arising, the nurses devised a behavior modification program that gave the patient more control over her currently ambiguous environment. The initial target behavior formulated was to reduce the number of times the patient put on her light. To achieve this goal, and to provide her with more control over her environment, the nurses devised a checklist on which all of the patient's treatments were listed (e.g., observation of tubes and drainage). Placed at her bedside, this checklist was made available to the patient. Each of the treatments that she received was recorded and, in addition, she was able to ask questions for one ten-minute session every two hours. At this time, a nurse would sit and talk with her. The procedure worked rapidly. Soon the patient reduced her demands and was able to sleep without interruption, for the first time. Thus, with the help of a simple procedure, both the nursing staff and the patient were able to resolve some of their problems. Providing a patient with some awareness of and some "control" over his treatment (e.g., a checklist) seems to be a worthwhile procedure for reducing the uneasiness that arises from being hospitalized recently.

In the first section of this part, it was mentioned that many patients can be taught behaviors pertinent to health maintenance, and that reinforcement for performing them derives from knowing

---

[25]Linda Harmon Aiken, "Patient problems are problems in learning," *American Journal of Nursing*, 70, No. 9, 1970, 1918.

that one is successfully caring for himself. Also, it was stated that *sometimes* this type of reinforcement is not potent enough. For some patients, therefore, specific procedures must be devised, at least in the beginning phases of health teaching, to help the patient to help himself. Thus, an individual with a coronary condition who must reduce his cigarette smoking may need more than instruction and encouragement. He may need to develop self-control. The methods involved in acquiring self-control are discussed in the Concluding Statement.

Many addictive behaviors, such as cigarette smoking, drinking excessive amounts of alcohol, or taking drugs, as well as other unhealthy activities, such as overeating, can be effectively and durably reduced through the acquisition of self-control. Curing various conditions of the stomach, heart, or kidney may depend on reducing these addictive behaviors. Other important ones, such as reading essential literature about routine health-care practices, systematically taking medications prescribed by the physician, or following a suitable diet can be increased through learning self-control. Various personal problems, such as arguing, also have proven amenable to self-regulatory procedures (e.g., Goldiamond, 1965).

The durability of changed behavior is enhanced because the individual becomes able to treat himself and gains control over the situations preventing him from effectively altering his own behavior. Self-control can be taught to the patient; that is, he can be taught behavior modification and can be allowed to develop for himself, the procedures necessary to bring his own behavior under control. The advantages of this teaching for handling relapses and for preventing future problems has already been mentioned.

Prevailing Sources of Behavior Modification

As indicated in Section 3.5, behavior modification is meaningful if the strengthened activities are relevant for the patient in his interactions with the environment. If the initial behaviors accelerated in treatment bring the patient into touch with existing sources of positive reinforcement in the natural environment, many new desirable social behaviors can be developed. This is because there exist in the environment naturally occurring behavior modification practices that shape many activities. If the patient can contact these sources of change, he can be helped to learn many new behaviors and to perpetuate ones already learned in the behavior modification program.

One approach to meaningfulness in altering behavior, therefore, is for the nurse to help the patient to make contact with other individuals who promote desirable behavior. To make this contact, the patient must be able to perform certain relevant behaviors, which the *other* individuals require.

Baer and Wolf (1967) have advanced the idea that the natural environment contains various sources of reinforcement which can be used for promoting extensive amounts of desirable social behavior in patients: They have called these natural sources of behavior modification, *communities of reinforcement.* According to the authors, many individuals can be helped if they are taught the behaviors which gain them entry into the communities of reinforcement. Thus, if a withdrawn and socially isolated child can be guided into just minimally interacting with his peers, the peer group, itself, can help the child develop. According to Baer and Wolf, the preschool situation is one community of reinforcement.

These investigators reported a project where an isolated four-year-old boy was initiated into his peer group at the preschool and, thereby, was able to develop many positive social relationships. Briefly, the child's teacher guided him into dealing with his classmates and reinforced him for this interaction. *Once the child had made contact with his peer group, however, the teacher's guidance and reinforcement became unnecessary.*

Before treatment began, the youngster would stare at the other children playing but would not participate; he did, however, follow the teachers around. To initiate contact between the child and his peer group, the teachers requested that the other children play with the boy. When these children initiated play, the teachers guided the child by literally telling him what to say and what to do. During each guided interaction, the teachers administered social reinforcers to the boy by praising him and by expressing much approval for his playing with the other children. The amount and frequency of this social reinforcement was reduced gradually (was made more intermittent). And when the teachers completely discontinued administering reinforcers for these minimal social behaviors, the activities did not decelerate. The child had made contact with his peers, and they helped him to extend and to perpetuate desirable social relationships.

Thus, the peer group can become agents of reinforcement, which makes generalization possible; that is, since the child's peers are present in many new situations and initiate many new behaviors, much widespread application can occur.

For many patients, desirable behavior can be made durable and generalization can occur, if the nurse can help to produce and to accelerate those *few behaviors* of the patient which gain him entry into some community of reinforcement. Once contact is made, a shift in reinforcement administration away from the nurse can take place eventually. The result will be many other desirable changes for the patient.

As Baer and Wolf point out, there are other communities of reinforcement, such as the language community, that can help make the results of a behavior modification program generalize. Consider, for example, a mental hospital patient who rarely interacts with others; that is, he is silent and unresponsive to the attempts of others to converse with him. Perhaps he may be helped if the nurse were to strengthen enough appropriate speech so that he could begin to converse with other coherent patients.

Similarly, it seems reasonable that a recently disabled patient can be helped during the early phases of rehabilitation, if interactions with others in the hospital or in the outside environment can be initiated. This initiation could avert the development of extreme dependency and withdrawal. For the recently ill, therefore, the objective of helping the patient to enter a community of other patients can begin during his stay in the hospital; the positive effects of such a contact can be maintained and can be developed by the community of patients in the hospital. When the patient leaves the hospital, this process can be extended into the outside environment, wherein other communities exist (an attempt to develop a special community of reinforcement for mental patients is discussed in Chapter 7 Section 7.2).

In sum, as shown in both Sections 3.5 and 3.6, there are several approaches for developing durable and generalized behavior changes. By making the schedule of reinforcement increasingly intermittent, by employing social reinforcers, by utilizing other helping agents, by teaching self-control, and by capitalizing on extant sources of behavior modification, nurses can make behavior modification programs meaningful, and prevention of behavior problems can become possible.

TERMS AND QUESTIONS

Terms

Community of reinforcement

Questions

1. How can the reinforcement practices of parents influence the prosocial behavior of children?
2. What are the advantages of teaching parents behavior modification?
3. What other helping agents, outside of the ones mentioned, may be enlisted by the nurse?
4. What relevance does behavior modification have for public-health nurses?
5. What are three target behaviors that must be strengthened in order to teach behavior modification to other helping agents?
6. How will you accelerate the cooperation of a patient whom you are teaching?
7. How will you teach the following individuals? Use the behavior modification technology.
   (a) arthritic patients about home-care behaviors pertinent to their illness;
   (b) a health-aide to change a dressing;
   (c) a mastectomy patient to perform exercises at home.
8. How will you teach behavior modification principles to the following persons?
   (a) a foster grandparent. The responsibility of this helping agent will be to teach a retarded child to feed himself.
   (b) a parent. The parent wants his eight-year-old boy to stop hitting his younger sister.

3.7 *USING THE NEGATIVE REINFORCEMENT PROCEDURE TO ACCELERATE BEHAVIOR*

This chapter has explained the important principles associated with accelerating desirable behavior through the Positive Reinforcement procedure. Positive Reinforcement describes *one contingent relationship between behavior and the environment* that can be used to strengthen behavior; that is, to strengthen behavior, one should change its consequences in such a way that pleasant events (e.g., money, food, and praise) become contingent on the behavior. The occurrence of the behavior has to produce the positive consequences.

In this context, therefore, *contingency* means that the positive reinforcer is administered *only if* the designated behavior occurs.

The relationship between behavior and its consequences may be arranged *purposely* or *accidentally* (e.g., you walk under a ladder, and you have a mishap).

Positive Reinforcement, as a method for accelerating desirable behavior, is a purposely arranged contingency. There are, in addition, three other ways that the relationship between behavior and its consequences can be arranged purposely; that is, a total four contingent relationships can be employed in behavior modification. Two are described in Chapter 4, along with another procedure called Extinction. Extinction involves the disruption of a contingency between a behavior and its consequence.

The contingent relationship that is the subject of this section *involves the removal or postponement of an unpleasant event contingent on the occurrence of some particular behavior.* More specifically, because its occurrence removes or postpones a punishing or unpleasant event, the behavior increases in frequency.

Reinforcers are events in the environment of a person that influence the frequency of his behavior. If a consequence increases the frequency of the behavior that it follows, the event is a positive reinforcer. *If an event increases the frequency of the behavior that removes or postpones it, the event is a negative reinforcer.* (In this text, when the term *reinforcer* is written alone, however, we mean positive reinforcer.) Negative reinforcers are unpleasant events for the individual. Many occurrences can function as negative reinforcers, such as a loud no from another person, uncomfortable climatic conditions, or the sight of something distasteful. *But* it is important to remember that these events can be called negative reinforcers only if they can affect the individuals behavior in a certain way—namely, if they can *increase the frequency of the behavior that removes or postpones them.*

A behavior modification program designed to accelerate a particular behavior by following its occurrence with the removal or postponement of an unpleasant event is using the *Negative Reinforcement procedure.*

To reiterate, the conditions of treatment can be arranged so that the behavior produces a positive reinforcer—this method is the Positive Reinforcement procedure. The conditions of treatment also can be arranged so that the behavior is followed by the removal or postponement of a negative reinforcer—this method is the Negative Reinforcement procedure. With both these operations, the consequences of the behavior (the removal or postponement of the negative reinforcer and the presentation of the positive reinforcer) are contingent on the occurrence of the behavior. Notice, with the Negative Reinforcement procedure, the word *negative* does not mean that the activity decreases. On the contrary, *both the Negative and the Positive Reinforcement procedures are used to accelerate behavior.*

To illustrate Negative Reinforcement, consider these examples. Suppose you dislike dogs and will go out of your way to avoid them. Also, let us suppose that you walk home each afternoon after work and realize that one block from your house a large great dane usually is playing outside. You can avoid passing by the dog if you take a detour that involves two additional blocks of walking. Therefore, you take this long way home each day. Your walking the extra distance (a behavior) is negatively reinforced because it avoids the dog (an unpleasant stimulus). Because the dog is a potent negative reinforcer, walking the extra distance, which avoids it, will occur regularly—it will be a strong behavior.

Apologizing in social situations is likely to occur, when this behavior will avoid social recrimination. Thus, if you were to step accidentally on someone's toes in a dark movie theater, you would be likely to say "excuse me," and so on. The strength of apologizing in circumstances such as this one is a function of its past effectiveness in avoiding unpleasant social responses from your victims.

Acquiescing to a child's nagging not only positively reinforces him but also negatively reinforces the parent; that is, by giving in, you can turn off the whining and the crying.

The interaction patterns of many married couples, at times, seem to be more related to conditions of negative than of positive reinforcement. A wife may cook elaborate meals because she doesn't want to listen to her husband complain. Conversely, a husband may fix things in the home, not so much because he wants to have things functioning efficiently but because he wants to avoid or to escape the recrimination and the complaining of his wife—this is negative reinforcement. A valuable approach in marriage counseling is aimed at strengthening mutual positive reinforcement and at reducing these other patterns of behavior (Stuart, 1969).

The Negative Reinforcement procedure can be used to accelerate desirable behavior, provided that the environment is arranged so that the occurrence of the activity removes or postpones some negative reinforcer. For example, to help a mother to improve her 8½-year-old son's behavior, Bernal et al. (1968) employed both Positive and Negative Reinforcement methods. (Only Negative Reinforcement will be explained here.) The child, for all intensive purposes, ruled the home; in fact, he often told his mother what she could and could not do. The mother, in turn, was completely inept at controlling her son, let alone at teaching him anything desirable. An important step in helping the mother to improve the boy's behavior was establishing her control as a mother. Therefore, she was instructed to follow her child's undesirable behavior (e.g., his refusal to obey requests and his use of inappropriate language) with cues denoting anger (e.g., saying "don't" angrily and frowning). If presenting them did not result in a reduction of the boy's abusive activities, he was to receive a spanking (see Aversive Stimulation in Section 4.1, Chapter 4).

Hints of indignation had never been consistently or systematically backed up by a punishing event, such as a spanking. Consequently, these cues were coupled with the spanking in order to increase their potency; that is, by coupling the anger cues with a spanking, in much the same way that praise can be coupled with a pleasant event (food), the effectiveness of the anger cues as unpleasant events (as negative reinforcers) was increased. In short, the threats were backed up.

After augmenting the mother's control in this manner, the desirable behaviors of the child became more frequent and his undesirable behavior became less frequent. More specifically, the desirable behaviors of the child that removed these anger cues became stronger due to the Negative Reinforcement procedure, and undesirable behaviors that lead to the presentation of these cues became weaker (Aversive Stimulation). As the behavior modification program proceeded, the number of spankings actually administered decreased. In addition, both mother and child expressed increased liking for one another; furthermore, the boy seemed to acquire more respect for his mother's authority. It should be mentioned that during treatment, the mother was given instructions, corrective feedback, and positive reinforcers in order that she might learn to help her child to behave more capably than before.

In sum, although Negative Reinforcement is not employed as frequently as Positive Reinforcement for accelerating desirable behavior, it may be useful, especially in combination with other methods. The treatment definition of Negative Reinforcement is as follows:

Negative Reinforcement is a procedure for increasing the frequency of a desired behavior by removing or by postponing an unpleasant event contingent on the occurrence of the activity. Thus, to remove (to escape from) the glare of the sun, you put on sunglasses; to postpone (to avoid) the sight of a dog, you travel out of your way; to avoid social recrimination, you apologize for a discourteous act. In these examples, putting on sunglasses, traveling out of your way, and apologizing are each behaviors that occur frequently because they either remove or postpone some undesired outcome. Negative Reinforcement requires that the nurse arrange the patient's environment in such a way that the occurrence of a desirablė behavior removes or postpones some unpleasant consequence. The result will be a strengthening of the wanted activity.

Application 8. Increasing the Regularity of Self-Administered Medication by Using the Negative Reinforcement Procedure

One of the major problems encountered in rehabilitating patients, notably geriatric ones, is inaccuracy in adhering to a medical regimen (Taylor and Gaitz, 1969). Being consistent and systematic in self-administering medicines, in particular, is a problem. Patients of various ages on oral medications often do not follow their instructions and may take their medications incorrectly (Hecht, 1970).

The purpose of the experiment described below (Azrin and Powell, 1969)[26] was to explore the effectiveness of several methods for promoting regularity in the self-administration of medicines. The healthy women, aged 20 to 33, who volunteered for this experiment were told that the pills, which they were to take every half-hour during the day, had no active ingredients. This study, therefore, was only a first attempt at understanding how to improve accuracy in self-medication. Future studies with actual patients who experience difficulty in consistently taking prescribed medications should be performed.

In this experiment, three procedures were compared; they were as follows:

1. *Taking pills from a container.* This method is similar to the usual manner in which people take pills; that is, a portable container was given to each woman, and she was instructed to take a pill every half hour.
2. *Taking pills after being signalled by an alarm timer.* This device was also a portable pill container. But it sounded a three-second hum when the woman was supposed to take her pill.

[26]N. H. Azrin and J. Powell, "Behavioral engineering: The use of response priming to improve prescribed self-medication," *Journal of Applied Behavior Analysis*, 2, 1969, 39–42.

In short, the container simply alerted each participant that it was time to administer her pill.

3. *Taking pills from a behaviorally engineered dispenser.* Similar to the alarm timer, this portable device sounded a hum when it was time to take a pill. The tone, however, could be shut off (removed) only if the knob on the dispenser was turned. Then the tone would cease—negative reinforcement—and a pill was ejected into the woman's hand; also, the timer on the dispenser was automatically reset for another half-hour.

Although having a pill in hand was no guarantee that the woman would swallow it, the authors found that once the woman was holding it, she would place it into her mouth. Notice that the tone of the dispenser could be shut off only if its knob was turned; this activity was negatively reinforced because it *removed* the tone. Specifically, the sound of the tone set the occasion for turning the knob, a behavior that was then negatively reinforced—it shut off the tone.

From the results, the superiority of this third approach—the "Behavioral Engineering" approach—was evident. With this procedure, most of the pills were self-administered at the appropriate time. The effectiveness of this method, which designates target behaviors and which utilizes devices such as the one described in this study, has been shown with other problems, for example, with poor posture (Azrin et al., 1968).

TERMS AND QUESTIONS

Terms

Negative reinforcer
Negative reinforcement procedure
Behavioral engineering

Questions

1. How will you design a behavior modification program using both the Positive and Negative Reinforcement procedures (in combination) for an ulcer patient? The goal is to increase the frequency of his following a prescribed diet.
2. How may you make an event into a potent negative reinforcer?

3.8 A SYNTHESIS

Chapter 3 has focused on how to accelerate an individual's relevant behavior in order to help him to act more capably. In this regard, all but one of the preceding parts have stressed the Positive Reinforcement procedure. The Negative Reinforcement procedure also has been discussed as one approach for accelerating desirable behavior. The elements that compose Positive Reinforcement have been described one at a time. This was done, *not* because positive reinforcement plans are simplistic but for purposes of clarity and understanding. Generally, the elements are combined in a behavior modification program (e.g., food and tokens are used together as are Instructing and Demonstration–Imitation techniques).

In addition, this chapter has put forth three requirements for behavior modification (e.g., relevance, effectiveness, and meaningfulness). They apply to all programs, regardless of whether the goal is to accelerate or to decelerate behavior; they are derived mainly from criteria proposed by Baer, Wolf and Risley (1968) and by Risley (1969).

The relevance requirement means that any behavior to be modified must be important to society and to the individual.

Effective behavior modification refers to changes extensive enough for one to say that the individual is acting significantly better. In other words, there must be sufficient improvement in the individual's behavior to enable him to function capably in accordance with society's requirements. Effective behavior modification in Chapter 3 involves marked increases in the frequency of desirable behavior. Effective behavior modification in the next chapter will be related to marked decreases in the frequency of undesirable behavior. The opinion that a program has been effective is often difficult to make because of the differing standards of the judges and because of their disagreements as to what society in fact requires. In the last analysis, according to Baer and his associates, the individuals having to deal with the behavior are the best judges of whether behavior modification has been effective. These judges can be the patient or the individuals responsible for his care.

Much of what has been discussed in Chapter 3 that is pertinent to the Positive Reinforcement procedure (e.g., defining goals into target behaviors and administering reinforcers contingently) is also related to the effective use of the Negative Reinforcement method. What follows is a reiteration of the basic principles necessary for effectively applying Positive Reinforcement to accelerate desirable behavior:

1. Accurately define, observe, and record the target behavior—the behavior to be accelerated. These three topics will be discussed more completely in Chapter 5.
2. Specify in advance where the Positive Reinforcement procedure will take place (e.g., the situations) and who the agents of reinforcement will be (e.g., the nurse or the family).
3. State what events will be employed as positive reinforcers:
   a. Ascertain what events can function as positive reinforcers for the patient. An event is a positive reinforcer only if it will increase the frequency of behavior that produces it.
   b. Use potent reinforcers; that is, use positive reinforcers that retain their power to strengthen for long periods. Primary, acquired, generalized-acquired, and activity reinforcers may be employed in the Positive Reinforcement procedure. Coupling generalized-acquired with activity reinforcers is particularly useful. Combining several potent reinforcers in a Positive Reinforcement procedure is suggested (e.g., reinforcer menu).
4. Explicitly designate the contingency between the target behavior and the positive reinforcers it produces—what are the particular consequences, for the individual, of performing the target behavior? The use of a behavioral contract is an interesting strategy which specifies contingencies.
5. If necessary, allow the person (especially a child) time to adjust to the situation where positive reinforcers will be dispensed and to the nurses who will be dispensing them.
6. Administer positive reinforcers immediately following the occurrence of the desired behavior.
7. Administer a balanced amount of reinforcement—neither too many nor too few positive reinforcers should be made contingent on behavior.
8. Administer positive reinforcers on a continuous schedule at first, but then make it intermittent. A continuous schedule is most efficient in the beginning phases of the Positive Reinforcement procedure, when the target behavior is being accelerated. Intermittent reinforcement (e.g., variable ratio or variable in-

terval) is most efficient in maintaining behavior once it has been accelerated. Intermittent schedules result in more durable behavior (a meaningful outcome).

9. Administer positive reinforcers, notably praise, sincerely.

In order to cause large increases in desirable behavior by using the Positive Reinforcement procedure, the behavior must take place occasionally. Many activities, however, almost never occur or occur so infrequently that administering positive reinforcers for them is almost impossible (see Application 6). In these situations, a combination of several behavior-producing techniques can be employed. They are the following: Shaping, Instructing, Demonstration–Imitation, Guiding and Fading, and Linking.

Meaningfulness, the last requirement for behavior modification programs that was discussed in this chapter, was explained mainly with reference to the facilitation of durable and general alterations. When the meaningfulness requirement is fulfilled, the possibility of preventing relapses and other problems from occurring becomes more likely. Preventative behavior modification, which was included in this discussion of meaningfulness, was associated primarily with using behavior modification to teach other helping agents health-care practices as well as behavior modification per se.

In the parts concerned with meaningful behavior modification, the following specific suggestions were made:

1. Incorporate techniques that are likely to result in durable and generalized behavior changes; that is, make the schedule of reinforcement gradually more intermittent, and establish the potency of social reinforcers. Social events, such as praise or attention from other people, can become positive reinforcers if coupled with events that are already powerful ones (e.g., food). Tokens also can be made into powerful reinforcers by using this same procedure.
2. Utilize behavior-modification principles to teach others (e.g., patients, health-aides, families, large groups) health-care practices. When these individuals master the procedures, there will result increased likelihood of long-range positive effects for the patient. Positive-reinforcement principles provide the nurse with a technology for effective and meaningful health teaching.
3. Utilize behavior-modification principles to teach other helping agents (e.g., families, school teachers, and foster grandparents) about behavior modification. This approach to meaningfulness,

possibly more than any other, is closest to fostering the prevention of behavior problems.

4. Teach the patient self-control.
5. Bring the patient into contact with existing sources of behavior modification, that is, with communities of reinforcement, by accelerating the required "entry" behaviors.

In sum, Chapter 3 has detailed how the Positive Reinforcement procedure can be applied *effectively* and *meaningfully* to *relevant* behaviors for promoting physical and mental health. No other method is as valuable as this one for the nurse to employ in helping individuals to behave more capably. In the next chapter, several ways of decelerating undesirable behavior will be presented; they are useful, especially when combined with Positive Reinforcement.

SUPPLEMENTARY READINGS

AYLLON, T., AND N. H. AZRIN "Reinforcement and Instructions with Mental Patients," *Journal of the Experimental Analysis of Behavior*, 7, 1964, 327–331.

BAER, D. M., R. F. PETERSON, AND J. A. SHERMAN "Building an Imitative Repetoire by Programming Similarity between Child and Model as Discriminative for Reinforcement," Paper read at biennial meeting of Society for Research in Child Development, Minneapolis, 1965.

BANDURA, A. *Principles of Behavior Modification*. New York: Holt, Rinehart & Winston, Inc., 1969, pp. 236–240.

BLACKHAM, G. J., AND A. SILBERMAN *Modification of Child Behavior*. Belmont, California: Wadsworth Publishing Company, Inc., 1971, pp. 28–30.

FERSTER, C. B., AND MARY C. PERROTT *Behavior Principles*. New York: Appleton-Century-Crofts, 1968, pp. 1–67.

LEBOW, M. D. "Behavior Modification for the Family," in *Family Therapy: An Introduction to Theory and Technique*, eds. G. Erickson and T. Hogan. Belmont, California: Brooks/Cole, 1972.

LOVAAS, O. I., B. SCHAEFFER, AND J. Q. SIMMONS "Building Social Behavior in Autistic Children by Use of Electric Shock," *Journal of Experimental Research in Personality*, 1, 1965, 99–109.

PATTERSON, G. R. "Behavioral Intervention Procedures in the Classroom and in the Home," in *Handbook of Psychotherapy and Behavior Change: An Empirical Analysis*, eds. A. E. Bergin and S. L. Garfield. New York: John Wiley & Sons, Inc., 1971.

PETERSON, R. F. "Imitation: A Basic Behavioral Mechanism," in *Operant Procedures in Remedial Speech and Language Training*, eds. H. N. Sloane, Jr., and Barbara D. Macauley. Boston: Houghton Mifflin Company, 1968.

REESE, ELLEN P. *The Analysis of Human Operant Behavior*. Dubuque: Wm. C. Brown Company, Publishers, 1966.

SKINNER, B. F. "The Technology of Teaching," *Proceedings of the Royal Society*, 162, 1965, 427–443. Also in B. F. Skinner, *The Technology of Teaching*. New York: Appleton-Century-Crofts, 1968.

STOLZ, STEPHANIE, AND M. M. WOLF "Visually Discriminated Behavior in a 'Blind' Adolescent Retardate," *Journal of Applied Behavior Analysis*, 2, 1969, 65–77.

THARP, R. G., AND R. J. WETZEL *Behavior Modification in the Natural Environment*. New York: Academic Press, 1969.

WAHLER, R. G. "Behavior Therapy for Oppositional Children: Love is Not Enough," Paper read at the meeting of the Eastern Psychological Association, Washington, April, 1968.

four *Decelerating Undesirable Behavior*

4.1 *A GENERAL STATEMENT*

As indicated in Chapter 1, there are essentially two reasons why the nurse labels a behavior objectionable and wishes to eliminate it or to reduce its strength. *The first reason is that she may consider the behavior itself undesirable.* For example, the patient may be engaging in self-mutilating behavior, as in the case of the self-destructive child; or he may be putting the lives of others in jeopardy, as in the case of the firebug; or he may be acting in a way that interferes with the effective management of the institution (e.g., stealing); or he may be acting in a "sick" manner (e.g., hallucinating).

The second reason why the nurse may consider the patient's behavior as basically undesirable has to do with how frequently, and in what situations, the behavior occurs, rather than with the content of the particular behavior per se. For example, discussing your problems is not undesirable in and of itself. Discussing your problems every time you have a listener, however, may get you the reputation of being a chronic complainer. The mental patient who seeks out the nurse to talk about "things" is behaving appropriately, but the patient who visits the nursing station 25 times a day is behaving unfittingly.

Whatever the reason for considering a patient's behavior undesirable, reducing or eliminating it not only will help him to act more capably but also will result in his being judged more competent and appropriate than before. It is difficult to label a patient's behavior without labeling the patient himself. Thus, a person who complains often is called a complainer and an individual who emits pathological statements, such as, "I'm the son of God," is called a schizophrenic. Consequently, by successfully reducing undesirable behavior, the nurse can alter society's judgment of the patient. Furthermore, by helping to eliminate unwanted behavior, the nurse creates the opportunity for the patient to experience greater positive reinforcement from society—reinforcement which society gives to its capable members. In addition, the patient is able to consider, more adequately, new behaviors that result in even greater benefits from society.

To influence society's evaluation of the patient by unburdening him of his behavior problems, the nurse will have to be an agent of effective treatment. If the nurse-practitioner is in continuous contact with the patient, the conditions for effective treatment are optimal—the optimal conditions exist for applying behavior-modification principles.

This chapter is concerned with those practices involved with the reduction or the elimination of undesirable behavior. Each of the procedures presented is used to reduce or to eliminate objectionable behavior, hence the term *deceleration*. Each, however, is different in its approach to this goal. This chapter will outline the definition and the use of the deceleration procedures, and the examples presented will illustrate their application in various settings.

Notice that before any of the methods can be successfully employed to change a patient's behavior, the nurse should ascertain the following:

1. *The undesirable behavior.* The specific behavior to be decelerated is the target behavior.
2. *The frequency of the undesirable behavior.* The number of times the behavior occurs in a minute, or an hour, or a day indicates its strength. By knowing how often a behavior occurs before treatment, the nurse can decide whether the behavior modification procedure employed is effective; that is, if the activity of the patient remains unchanged when the method is implemented, it is inappropriate for the specific patient (see Chapter 5).
3. *The situations in which the undesirable behavior occurs.* This

information involves knowing where the patient is likely to engage in the undesirable behavior and when this activity will occur.

Each of the deceleration procedures is presented individually for purposes of explanation; combining them with the Positive Reinforcement method discussed in the previous chapter, however, is strongly advised (see Section 4.8).

QUESTIONS

1. What are the reasons for judging a behavior undesirable?
2. What information should you gather before implementing a deceleration procedure?

4.2 *AVERSIVE STIMULATION*

Description and Treatment Definition

When a behavior, such as touching a hot stove, is decreased because something painful has followed it, the situation is generally described as punishing. The events which take place after this behavior, such as being burned, are termed *aversive*; when a distasteful occurrence takes place after an activity, it usually is less likely to happen again. For example, suppose that a mother, while standing by her livingroom window, observes her three-year-old son run into the street to retrieve a ball. Frightened at the prospect of her son being hit by an oncoming car, she rushes toward him and spanks him harshly while she shouts, "Don't run into the street ever again." The child immediately responds by crying. Later in the day, he runs into the street again and once more receives the spanking and verbal reprimand. The next day the child's ball rolls into the street; but this time he tells his mother, and she retrieves it for him.

In this example, the child engaged in the behavior of running into the street, which his mother considered potentially harmful to his safety. To eliminate the undesirable activity and to prevent it from happening again, the mother spanked and scolded her child. The spanking and the scolding events are *aversive stimuli* that the child received from the mother. These stimuli had two observable effects. First, they elicited crying in the child (respondent behavior); second, *because both these stimuli (spanking and scolding) were presented after the child's behavior (running into the street) had occurred, it was less likely to occur in the future.* Remember, the child did not run into the street the next day when his ball rolled there.

To reiterate, spanking and scolding are stimuli that followed the child's running into the street (a behavior). Because the presentation of these stimuli were contingent on the occurrence of his running into the street, this behavior decreased in strength; that is, the child did not run into the street the next day in order to retrieve his ball. The activity became less probable.

Presenting an aversive stimulus when some response or behavior occurs in order to reduce the frequency of that behavior is called the *Aversive Stimulation* procedure. This describes the third contingent relationship. The first two contingent relationships, described by the Positive Reinforcement and Negative Reinforcement procedures, are employed in accelerating behavior. Aversive Stimulation is used in decelerating behavior.

With Negative Reinforcement, a behavior may be *increased* in frequency if the removal or postponement of an unpleasant event (negative reinforcer) were made contingent on the occurrence of the behavior. With Aversive Stimulation, a behavior can be *decreased* in frequency if its occurrence results in the presentation of an unpleasant event; that is, if the unpleasant event (aversive stimulus) is presented contingent on the occurrence of the behavior. (The terms *aversive stimulus* and *negative reinforcer* both describe unpleasant events. To magnify the difference between Negative Reinforcement and Aversive Stimulation, however, both these terms have been put forth to describe disagreeable occurrences; but no difference, in this text, exists between saying that an aversive stimulus is presented or that a negative reinforcer is presented.) The treatment definition of Aversive Stimulation is as follows:

Aversive Stimulation is a procedure in which a painful or unpleasant event such as a verbal reprimand, shock, or noise is presented contingent on the occurrence of an undesirable behavior. The major effect of the Aversive Stimulation procedure is to decelerate behavior.

Additional Comments

As a method for decelerating undesirable behavior, Aversive Stimulation is effective. It is worthwhile for applying to many problems (Baer, 1970), but unpleasant side effects may result from its use (Bandura, 1969, pp. 308–13); these side effects are most likely to occur when only Aversive Stimulation is employed for treating the patient.

One of these potential undesired side effects is that the patient avoids either the situation in which the aversive stimulus is presented or the nurse presenting the aversive stimulus, or both. Thus, in much the same way that nurses who administer positive reinforcers can become reinforcers, nurses who administer aversive stimuli can become aversive to the patient. And he may learn behaviors which avoid or remove these agents, such as running away from or becoming aggressive against them (Negative Reinforcement).

The question of whether to use Aversive Stimulation for decelerating undesirable behavior should be rephrased into how best can this procedure be employed, that is, how can it be used with a maximum of desired effects and with a minimum of undesired side effects? The answer to this question, in general, involves making sure that the aversive stimulus is, in fact, aversive, administering it immediately following the occurrence of the undesirable behavior, and administering it on a continuous schedule (i.e., each occurrence of the undesirable behavior should be followed by the aversive stimulus).

Most important to minimizing the unwanted side effects, especially the avoidance of the nurses, is to combine the Aversive Stimulation and Positive Reinforcement procedures. The nurse who administers aversive stimuli contingent on undesirable behavior should also administer positive reinforcers contingent on desirable behavior. Furthermore, if the accelerated desirable behavior is incompatible with the undesirable behavior that is followed by the aversive stimulus, the reduction of this unwanted behavior will be facilitated. (See Section 4.7.)

Application 9. Using Aversive Stimulation for Treating a Self-Destructive Child

This example of the Aversive Stimulation procedure (Tate and Baroff, 1966)[1] illustrates its application in treating a nine-year-old self-destructive and retarded boy. In order to give a clear understanding of the behavior problem involved, the authors' description of this patient, Sam, will be presented.

---

[1]B. G. Tate and George S. Baroff, "Aversive control of self-injurious behavior in a psychotic boy," *Behaviour Research and Therapy*, 4, 1966, 281–287.

> Sam was a nine-year-old, blind male who was transferred for evaluation and treatment on a research basis from an out-of-state psychiatric hospital to Murdoch Center, a state institution for the mentally retarded. At the age 5 he was diagnosed as autistic and was hospitalized. For the next 4 years he received group and individual psychotherapy, and drug therapy with no long-term benefit. Drugs were used in an effort to control self-injurious behavior, screaming, and hyperactivity.
>
> The SIB [self-injurious behavior] began at about the age of four and consisted of face slapping. By age nine, his SIB [self-injurious behavior] repertoire included banging his head forcefully against floors, walls, and other hard objects, slapping his face with his hands, punching his face and head with his fists, hitting his shoulder with his chin, and kicking himself. Infrequently he would also pinch, bite, and scratch others.
>
> At age eight, bilateral cataracts, a complete detachment of the left retina, and partial detachment of the right retina were discovered. An opthalmologist has suggested that the cataracts were probably congenital but were not noticed until they matured and that the retinal detachments were likely caused by head banging. The cataract in the right eye was removed soon after its discovery, leaving Sam with some light-dark vision and possibly some movement perception.
>
> Upon arrival at Murdoch Center, Sam was assigned a room in the infirmary and drugs were immediately discontinued. Casual observations were made for the first two weeks while he was adapting to his new environment. Following the adaptation period, eighteen 30-minute daily observation periods were conducted during which a female research assistant held Sam, tried to interest him in games, and ignored all SIR [self-injurious responses].[2]

Because the child was endangering his right retina by banging his head, an Aversive Stimulation procedure was employed (an aversive stimulus was made to follow his self-destructive behavior). The Aversive Stimulation method consisted of shock (the aversive stimulus) being delivered when each self-destructive behavior occurred. Thus, each time the child slapped his face or banged his head, he was given a half-second electric shock on his lower right leg. The stimulus was presented by touching him with a prod. Most of the

---

[2]Ibid., pp. 281–282.

time, the shock was administered immediately after the behavior had occurred, but sometimes, when the therapists were in another room, the shock was presented thirty- to thirty-five seconds later. In this study, the delay did not seem to interfere with the results.

On the first day of treatment, after Sam was observed for twenty-four minutes, he was instructed that a painful shock would be delivered when he hit himself. On this day, the Aversive Stimulation procedure lasted for two ninety-minute periods; it was found that Sam's self-injurious behavior decreased from what it had been prior to the implementation of this method. The authors stated that although shock did startle Sam, he did not cry. On the second day of treatment, Sam was left unrestrained for 5½ hours during which time he made 20 self-injurious responses, each one followed by shock. On the third day, Sam was left unrestrained for 8½ hours and made only 15 self-injurious responses. According to the authors' last report, 167 days had passed since the Aversive Stimulation procedure had been started. No self-injurious behaviors had occurred during the last twenty of these days. Also, they said Sam was free from bed most of the day, was participating in several activities and generally was more responsive.

In sum, the elements of this procedure were as follows:

1. An extremely undesirable class of target behaviors, that is, self-injurious responses were observed and recorded.
2. An Aversive Stimulation procedure was employed—each self-injurious behavior was followed by shocking the child.
3. The self-injurious behavior was found to decrease gradually until eventually it was eliminated.

Undoubtedly, the procedure used in this example was painful to the child. Nevertheless, it had fewer disastrous consequences for him than did his self-destructive behavior. Indeed, it would be far more punitive to allow Sam to beat himself to death, or to keep him restrained in his bed for many years than to subject him to the Aversive Stimulation procedure. By suppressing Sam's extremely dangerous behavior, through Aversive Stimulation, the therapists could positively reinforce many appropriate noninjurious activities. This chance may be one of the most important benefits of using Aversive Stimulation; that is, by suppressing frequently occurring undesirable behavior, the nurse will have the opportunity to positively reinforce desirable behavior.

TERMS AND QUESTIONS

Terms

Aversive stimuli

Aversive Stimulation procedure

Questions

1. What contingency does the Aversive Stimulation procedure involve?
2. What is the difference between the Aversive Stimulation and Negative Reinforcement methods?
3. Do you believe that Aversive Stimulation is unethical in all situations? If not, where do you think that it is appropriate?

4.3 *WITHDRAWAL OF POSITIVE REINFORCEMENT*

Description and Treatment Definition

Withdrawal of Positive Reinforcement is a procedure in which something appealing is taken away from or denied a person because he engages in an undesirable behavior. Suppose that in our initial example of the Aversive Stimulation method, in which the mother spanked and scolded her child for running into the street, she instead removed him from the play situation by taking him into the house. This method also might have resulted in the child no longer chasing his ball into the street. This deceleration procedure, however, is different from Aversive Stimulation in one essential way. With Aversive Stimulation, something distasteful, such as a slap, is presented following the occurrence of the undesirable behavior. With the Withdrawal of Positive Reinforcement, however, some positive (pleasant) stimulus is removed following the occurrence of the behavior.

Aversive Stimulation presents something aversive contingent on the occurrence of the behavior, whereas Withdrawal of Positive Reinforcement removes something pleasant contingent on the occurrence of the behavior. This method provides the fourth contingent relationship. With Positive Reinforcement, a behavior can be *increased* in frequency if the presentation of a positive reinforcer is made contingent on the occurrence of the activity. In contrast, with Withdrawal of Positive Reinforcement, a behavior can be *decreased* in frequency if its occurrence results in the withdrawal of a positive reinforcer, that is, the positive reinforcer is withdrawn contingent on the occurrence of the behavior.

The mother in our example took the child away from his enjoyable play activities and, thereby, immediately withdrew positive reinforcers. If the child were older, the mother could have taken away other reinforcers not actually present in the situation. The tardy behavior of a 15-year-old boy, who stays out too late on weeknights, for instance, may be reduced by withdrawing his weekend privileges (e.g., going to a basketball game). Of course, the adolescent should be made aware of this contingency in advance—staying out late on weeknights results in the forfeiture of weekend activities. The delayed withdrawal of a positive reinforcer may be effective, but more immediate revocation is recommended. Thus, subtracting points, for example, as soon as an undesirable behavior has occurred is preferable to delayed withdrawal of some selected activity reinforcer. The subtraction of points will have the desired results if they are positive reinforcers (e.g., a certain amount of these points may be required for the opportunity to engage in the activity reinforcer). The treatment definition of Withdrawal of Positive Reinforcement is as follows:

Withdrawal of Positive Reinforcement is a procedure in which a positive reinforcer is removed, denied, or ended contingent on the occurrence of an undesirable behavior.

A patient in a mental hospital, for example, may be instructed that whenever he steals food from others at meal times, his dessert will be withdrawn or simply not given to him.

Two Variants of the Withdrawal of Positive Reinforcement Procedure (Time-Out and Response-Cost)

Both *Time-Out* and *Response-Cost* are procedures in which a positive reinforcer is removed contingent on the occurrence of a behavior; both of these procedures are used to decelerate behavior. With Time-Out, the individual is either removed from a reinforcing situation for a period of time (e.g., he is isolated), or he remains physically in the situation and encounters a complete, but temporary, cessation of positive reinforcers (e.g., the nurse may turn away from the child for 20 seconds). With Response-Cost, the individual is given or has access to a pool of positive reinforcers, but each time he behaves undesirably, some of these reinforcers are withdrawn. Taking the individual away from reinforcing situations (Time-Out) has the same effect as taking positive reinforcers away from the individual (Response-Cost).

TIME-OUT. This method is the most frequently used Withdrawal of Positive Reinforcement procedure. Time-Out is always contingent on some specified undesirable behavior and is applicable to adult patients in mental hospitals, to delinquents, and to children with various types of problems. The length of the Time-Out periods may vary from short durations of a few seconds to long ones of many minutes. The optimal Time-Out to use is not known, but periods over 20 minutes should be employed with caution.

Time-Out has been applied effectively for decelerating the undesirable behavior of children living at home. In one reported study (Zeilberger, Sampen, and Sloane, 1968), for example, the mother of a 4½-year-old boy was instructed to place him in a room devoid of reinforcers when he was aggressive. When the child acted in these undesirable ways, she placed him in a time-out room for two minutes. In addition, the mother was told not to let her son out until two minutes of no undesirable behavior had elapsed. It is often necessary to extend the period, by 30 seconds, for example, to ensure that the individual is not removed from time-out when he is behaving undesirably. This extension is termed *time-out delay.*

It is also desirable not to argue with or lecture the person being placed in time-out, although the reasons for using this method should be given briefly.

Finally, it is necessary to caution that time-out can function as a *positive reinforcer strengthening undesirable behavior that results in it.* For instance if a child is involved in a situation which is not positively reinforcing, as are some hospital activities or classes at school, the withdrawal of the situation contingent on undesirable behavior, that is, the *presentation of time-out,* may be a positive reinforcer. In this case, the child will do all he can to cause the time-out to occur—he will behave undesirably. Obviously, this circumstance is unwanted.

RESPONSE-COST. Response-Cost, as stated, involves the subtraction of positive reinforcers from an individual's pool of available reinforcers; this subtraction is contingent on the person's performance of the undesired behavior. Holland (1969), for example, used Response-Cost as one of several procedures for reducing the times a seven-year-old boy set fires; more specifically, the author employed Response-Cost to decelerate the boy's match-striking behavior. The boy's father was told to place 20 pennies (positive reinforcers) beside a pack of matches and to inform his son of this contingency: Each match struck would result in one penny subtracted from the pile. The boy's match-striking quickly was decelerated.

Engeln et al. (1968) administered positive reinforcers, points redeemable for various material reinforcers, to two brothers contingent on appropriate behavior. The therapists used Response-Cost to decelerate the boys' aggressive behaviors; that is, they subtracted points from each child's accumulation contingent on his acting aggressively.

Additional Comments

When applied appropriately, Withdrawal of Positive Reinforcement is, indeed, an effective deceleration procedure. For correct use, the object withdrawn or the situation from which the individual is removed must function as a positive reinforcer. In addition, the withdrawal of the positive reinforcer should be contingent on the occurrence of the undesired behavior and should take place on a continuous schedule (i.e., each occurrence of the undesirable behavior should result in the withdrawal of the reinforcer). For most patients, Time-Out and Response-Cost should be administered *immediately* following the unwanted target behavior; but a delayed withdrawal of positive reinforcers can, in some instances, be effective. For children, however, immediate consequences are recommended over delayed ones. When Time-Out is used, it is important to end it only when the patient is behaving desirably, not undesirably; a time-out delay period may be necessary, especially in the early phases of the behavior modification program.

The Withdrawal of Positive Reinforcement procedure is not associated with the unwanted side effects (e.g., avoidance behavior) which are potentially possible with the Aversive Stimulation procedure. In fact, Time-Out has been used as part of an approach for increasing the reinforcement value of parents for their children (Wahler, 1969). In combination with Positive Reinforcement, Withdrawal of Positive Reinforcement is extremely valuable for helping individuals to behave more capably.

Application 10. Using the Withdrawal of Positive Reinforcement Procedure for Treating a Neurological Patient

This example (Barrett, 1962)[3] illustrates the effective application of Withdrawal of Positive Reinforcement for decelerating the spasmodic tics of a neurology patient. The author's description of the patient is reported below:

> The patient in this experiment was a 38-year-old veteran, hospitalized in the Neurology Service of a local Veterans Administration hospital. His extensive multiple tics started approximately 14 years ago, during his term of duty in the armed services. Although a medical discharge was available to him, the patient chose to continue in the service, eventually serving overseas, until regular discharge. Since then, he has been employed as an accountant by a single firm.
>
> An interview prior to the experiment revealed that the patient knew of no traumatic experience preceding the abrupt onset of tics. He told of awakening during the night with a choking sensation accompanied by a momentary inability to breathe or swallow. He recalled this as a frightening experience and was puzzled by the subsequent development of tics. Within a few months, spasmodic movements had developed in much of his body. At the time of this experiment, his major movements included contractions of neck, shoulder, chest, and abdominal muscles, head nodding, bilateral eye blinking, opening of the mouth, and other comparatively mild facial movements. The patient complained of difficulty in swallowing, hence of slow ingestion. His clear, intelligent speech was marked only occasionally by barely noticeable hesitation. . . .
>
> The patient had undergone psychological counseling for a number of months and had received pharmacological treatment which included a variety of tranquilizing and muscle-relaxing drugs. Neither treatment had afforded symptomatic relief. The patient displayed no outstanding symptoms of psychopathology. His tics were considered symptomatic of an extrapyramidal system disturbance and untreatable by conventional methods.
>
> Since he had experienced no success with other methods, the patient was highly motivated to participate in this experiment. Although he was soon discharged to return to work in a neighbor-

[3]Beatrice H. Barrett, "Reduction in rate of multiple tics by free operant conditioning methods," *Journal of Nervous and Mental Disease*, 135, 1962, 187–195.

ing state, he voluntarily rehospitalized himself two months later for continuation of the experiment.[4]

During treatment, the patient sat in a chair specially designed for recording each of his tics (the target behavior) and had to wear earphones, through which he could hear taped music. Since the interview information revealed that the patient enjoyed music (music was a positive reinforcer), he was allowed to select tapes which he especially liked. Each time he emitted a tic, the music he was listening to was interrupted for 1½ seconds. Therefore, each tic was followed by the withdrawal of a positive reinforcer; that is, each tic led to the interruption of ongoing positive reinforcement for a brief period of time.

In addition to Withdrawal of Positive Reinforcement, Aversive Stimulation was used. In this condition, unpleasant noise was presented through the earphones for 1½ seconds each time the patient twitched. When he did not do so for at least 1½ seconds, the noise stopped. Other investigators have found noise a productive consequence for decelerating undesirable behavior.

Both Withdrawal of Positive Reinforcement and Aversive Stimulation were effective in decelerating the patient's tics. Withdrawal of Positive Reinforcement, however, resulted in the greatest decrease in the behavior. In addition, with this procedure, many long tic-free intervals were observed.

In her discussion, Barrett suggested that Withdrawal of Positive Reinforcement and Aversive Stimulation procedures could be combined in the following manner: each tic could be followed by noise (Aversive Stimulation); if the patient did not emit a tic for a certain period of time, he could be positively reinforced by music (Positive Reinforcement); when the next tic occurred, music could be withdrawn (Withdrawal of Positive Reinforcement, and noise could be presented (Aversive Stimulation). As indicated previously, definite advantages result from combining behavior modification procedures.

In sum, Withdrawal of Positive Reinforcement—the removal of music contingent on the occurrence of tics—was employed effectively for a neurology patient.

Although this procedure yielded better results than Aversive Stimulation in this example, the results do not prove that Withdrawal of Positive Reinforcement always will be superior. Different patients with varying problems may require diverse procedures, and

---

[4]Ibid., pp. 187–188.

often several approaches are attempted before an effective one is found. A firm understanding of behavior modification methods will help you decide which one or which combination to employ.

TERMS AND QUESTIONS

Terms

Withdrawal of positive reinforcement procedure
Time-out
Time-out delay
Response-cost

Questions

1. How can Time-Out itself function as a positive reinforcer for a particular behavior and, thereby, be inappropriate for decelerating that behavior?
2. What is a major procedural difference between Response-Cost and Time-Out?
3. How can you employ the Withdrawal of Positive Reinforcement procedure to reduce the self-injurious behaviors of the child discussed in Application 9? (The authors of this study did, in fact, use a Time-Out method before they employed Aversive Stimulation.)
4. What are the four *contingent relationships* described in this book?

4.4 *SATIATION*

Description and Treatment Definition

As discussed in Chapter 3, Section 3.2, satiation is a process affecting the potency of a reinforcer. Satiation acts to reduce its potency, whereas deprivation acts to increase it.

Satiation can be used as a behavior modification procedure for reducing the strength of some undesired behavior. If an activity is followed by or is associated with too much positive reinforcement, it will decrease in frequency. Although satiation rarely is used on purpose in the everyday environment, it undoubtedly takes place anyway. As mentioned in Chapter 3, if you sit down at the dinner table to eat because you are hungry, and you begin eating your favorite foods, you probably will stop soon after you reach the point when you are hungry no longer; this result may occur even though a variety of your preferred dishes remain on the table. The strength of your eating behavior has been decreased, because you have ingested enough food; that is, you have had enough food to cause you to stop eating, at least temporarily.

If a specific food is eaten to excess after the point at which it is no longer desired, however, it is possible that you will lose *your taste for it* for a time and will not elect to consume it when you are hungry again. In both cases, eating behavior has been decelerated because it has been followed by *too much* positive reinforcement. Since eating is necessary for survival, it will be reduced only temporarily. Overeating a specific food, however, may result in a prolonged distaste for it.

In contrast to Aversive Stimulation and Withdrawal of Positive Reinforcement, Satiation, involves no contingent relationship between a behavior and the events following it. With Satiation, large amounts of the reinforcer are presented to the patient but not necessarily contingent on the occurrence of the undesirable activity; this procedure will be clarified in Application 11. The treatment definition of Satiation is as follows:

Satiation is a procedure in which large quantities of a positive reinforcer (usually related to the undesirable behavior) are made available to the patient until the undesirable behavior decreases.

For example, if the patient is hoarding printed matter, large amounts of it are given to him until he acquires so much that he stops hoarding it. Hoarding printed material is the undesirable behavior, and printed material, in this case, may be considered to be a positive reinforcer. When the patient is given large quantities of this reinforcer, his hoarding is likely to be reduced. In effect, he will "lose his taste" for the printed matter and will stop accumulating it. Therefore, the essential feature of Satiation is that one type of positive reinforcer (e.g., literature) is administered to the patient for an *extended period of time* or in *very large amounts* until the event becomes unpleasant; when this goal is reached, the undesirable behavior, which is associated with it, will be decelerated.

Additional Comments

Satiation can be applied effectively for reducing various behavior problems (e.g., hoarding, smoking, or eating an unbalanced diet).

But the procedure has not been extensively investigated in clinical situations. Consequently, no statement will be made about any potential undesirable side effects.

Its simplicity is one of its greatest advantages. As indicated below, Satiation may be employed productively.

Application 11. Using the Satiation Procedure in a Mental Hospital

In the following example (Ayllon, 1963),[5] Satiation was used to reduce the hoarding behavior of a schizophrenic patient, described by the author as follows:

> The patient was a 47-year-old female patient diagnosed as a chronic schizophrenic. The patient had been hospitalized for 9 years. Upon studying the patient's behavior on the ward, it became apparent that the nursing staff spent considerable time caring for her. In particular, there were three aspects of her behavior which seemed to defy solution. The first was stealing food. The second was the hoarding of the ward's towels in her room. The third undesirable aspect of her behavior consisted in her wearing excessive clothing, e.g., a half-dozen dresses, several pairs of stockings, sweaters, and so on.
>
> In order to modify the patient's behavior systematically, each of these three types of behavior (stealing food, hoarding, and excessive dressing) was treated separately.[6]

Only the hoarding problem will be considered here. Although the nurses had attempted to discourage this behavior, it, nevertheless, continued. Consequently, the nurses were forced to remove towels from the patient's room about twice a week.

To eliminate the patient's towel-hoarding activity (target behavior), the nurses first observed and recorded that at any given time she had stored approximately 19 to 29 towels in her room; then, they began placing more towels in her room. Specifically, the nurses instituted a Satiation procedure in which they *stopped removing towels from the patient's room and, instead, began giving her additional ones on a noncontingent basis,* that is, the patient received towels regardless of her behavior.

During the first week of the program, the nurses gave the pa-

---

[5]Teodoro Ayllon, "Intensive treatment of psychotic behaviour by stimulus satiation and food reinforcement," *Behaviour Research and Therapy*, 1, 1963, 53–61.

[6]Ibid., p. 54.

tient approximately 7 towels a day. But, by the third week, this figure had increased to 60 towels a day. In other words, towels were believed to be positively reinforcing hoarding, since the patient made every effort to acquire them. Once she was provided with an overabundance of towels, it was hoped that she would stop accumulating them.

This hope was realized. When the number of towels in the patient's room reached 625, she began to remove them, herself. Once this activity occurred, the nurses stopped giving the patient the unnecessary towels. During the following year, only about one or two could be found in her room at any given time. Thus, hoarding was eliminated permanently after the Satiation program ended, and no undesirable behavior was substituted—there was no "symptom substitution."

According to the author, after the number of towels in the patient's room reached 625, continued hoarding became unpleasant. Consequently, she began to remove them. Her interesting remarks during the Satiation program, which reflect the change in her feelings about the towels, are presented below:

> During the first few weeks of satiation, the patient was observed patting her cheeks with a few towels, apparently enjoying them. Later, the patient was observed spending much of her time folding and stacking the approximately 600 towels in her room. A variety of remarks were made by the patient regarding receipt of towels. All verbal statements made by the patient were recorded by the nurse. The following represent typical remarks made during this experiment. First week: As the nurse entered the patient's room carrying a towel, the patient would smile and say, "Oh, you found it for me, thank you." Second week: When the number of towels given to the patient increased rapidly, she told the nurses, "Don't give me no more towels. I've got enough." Third week: "Take them towels away. . . . I can't sit here all night and fold towels." Fourth and fifth weeks: "Get these dirty towels out of here." Sixth week: After she had started taking the towels out of her room, she remarked to the nurse, "I can't drag any more of these towels, I just can't do it."[7]

In sum, by presenting large quantities of the positive reinforcer (towels) to the patient throughout the day, the nurses were able to decelerate her bothersome behavior.

---

[7]Ibid., p. 57.

Rehabilitating behavior problems such as this one, which prevent the individual from capably living in the community, should be one goal of a behavior modification program.

TERMS AND QUESTIONS

Terms

Satiation procedure

Questions

1. Both the Aversive Stimulation and the Satiation procedures *present* events (stimuli) in order to reduce undesirable behavior. How do these stimuli and these procedures differ?
2. How will you design a behavior modification program using Satiation for decelerating cigarette smoking?

4.5 *EXTINCTION*

Description and Treatment Definition

This method, a very effective behavior modification procedure, is one in which the positive reinforcers that have followed the occurrence of a behavior are discontinued. The result is to decrease the frequency of the behavior. In other words, if an activity occurs very often because it is followed by positive reinforcers, and these reinforcers are discontinued, the behavior will occur less often and perhaps eventually will be eliminated.

Consider, for example, a mental patient in a large hospital who resists going to sleep at night and as part of his routine continually complains to the nurses about his hallucinations. He has to be told six or seven times to get ready for bed, and, once in bed, he will complain that he is unable to sleep because strange odors are permeating the ward. Since no one else can detect them, it is assumed that the patient is hallucinating the smells. In addition, let us suppose that this patient engages in the undesirable behaviors each night for an hour or two before he goes to sleep. The nurses respond by informing him that it is bedtime, by listening to his complaints, and at times by telling him that they do not detect the odors. In short, the nurses rarely ignore the patient's behavior but instead pay attention to it or, more accurately, provide attention for it.

Eventually, the nurses may decide that these bothersome activities must cease. Consequently, they tell the patient to go to bed only once and resolve that they will no longer pay attention to his nighttime complaints. After several nights of staying up late and complaining (perhaps even more than usual), the patient goes to bed and falls asleep after being told to do so only once. On future occasions, the nurses observe that the patient retires on time and only rarely complains about odors.

Initially, attention from the nurses followed the patient's complaints, and the grumbling as well as other difficulties occurred frequently, suggesting that attention from the nurses probably was perpetuating the patient's undesirable nighttime routine. The nurses' indulgence was not necessarily the original cause of the activity however. Proof that attention from the nurses was perpetuating the problem behavior is shown in part by the decrease in the patient's complaining when attention no longer followed it (i.e., when the nurses ignored his complaints).

In other words, attention from the nurses was positively reinforcing the patient's resistance to going to bed and his complaints about odors. When the positive reinforcer following a behavior is discontinued, that is, when it no longer takes place after the behavior, the procedure is called Extinction. As a result of Extinction, the activity diminishes in frequency. Since a positive reinforcer has been discontinued or has been removed, the method used is referred to most accurately, as *Extinction of positively reinforced behavior*. It is possible also to extinguish *negatively reinforced* behavior, but the operations are more complex than these (see Bandura, 1969, pp. 385–414).

As indicated in Chapter 3, Extinction involves the disruption of a contingency. Extinction of positively reinforced behavior means that the positive reinforcer previously contingent on the behavior has been discontinued. Thus, if a high school student's perpetual hand raising in class is being followed by notice from the teacher, discontinuing this attention will result in a decrease of the hand-raising behavior. In other words, the contingency between hand raising and teacher attention is disrupted. The treatment definition of Extinction of positively reinforced behavior is as follows:

Extinction, as it applies to positively reinforced behavior, is a procedure in which the positive reinforcers that have followed the occurrence of the behavior are discontinued.

For example, if attention, whether in the form of praise or of reproof, is following a frequently occurring behavior, it probably is a positive reinforcer for the activity. Extinction will take place if attention is discontinued (if it no longer follows the occurrence of the behavior). The result of Extinction is a decrease in the frequency of the behavior. In short, if an activity is *no longer* followed by positive reinforcers, its frequency will become decelerated.

Additional Comments

A great deal of evidence exists to prove the effectiveness of Extinction. It works well in many situations and for various problems. If an unwanted behavior is occurring frequently, and the nurse can ascertain what events probably are reinforcing it, these occurrences should be removed. A very common Extinction procedure, applicable to decelerating undesirable social behavior (e.g., tantruming) maintained by attention, is to simply *ignore* the activity. Thus, in the example of the child who scratched herself excessively, referred to in the previous chapter (see Section 3.5 of Chapter 3), the mother was told to ignore the scratching by not providing *any* attention for it.

Extinction does not have the potential unwanted side effects of Aversive Stimulation and does not require the *contingent* removal of a positive reinforcer as does Withdrawal of Positive Reinforcement; with Extinction, the reinforcers simply are discontinued.

It is extremely important, however, to be *consistent* in discontinuing reinforcers. If some of the occurrences of the undesired behavior are occasionally reinforced, it will be more difficult to decelerate. Recall that a behavior is less likely to be decelerated when an intermittent schedule of reinforcement is or has been operating; occasionally administering reinforcers for a behavior is equivalent to intermittently reinforcing it. Thus, to decelerate a behavior effectively by Extinction, the positive reinforcer must be discontinued *completely* and must no longer follow any occurrence of the behavior.

In the beginning phases of Extinction, an increase in the undesirable behavior may occur, but this effect will be only temporary. It is most likely to happen if the schedule of positive reinforcement was continuous. But the behavior will decelerate more rapidly if it was reinforced continuously rather than intermittently; intermittent schedules produce durable behavior, that is, behavior which resists deceleration once reinforcement is completely discontinued.

Finally, it is important to mention that when Extinction of unwanted behavior is combined with Positive Reinforcement of desirable behavior in one treatment program, the results are more likely to be long lasting. This combination of procedures is one of the most useful strategies for the nurse to employ.

Application 12. Using Extinction to Reduce Undesirable Behavior for a Retarded Child

There are numerous examples of adults and children being treated with Extinction procedures. The following case study (Wolf et al., 1965)[8] shows how the tantrum and vomiting behaviors of a retarded child were reduced by applying Extinction.

In this case study, the patient (Laura) was a nine-year-old retarded girl with cerebral palsy. Laura's dormitory nurse stated that fairly regularly, the child would vomit immediately after her admission to the institution but after awhile this practice had declined. When Laura was placed in a classroom at the institution, however, her undesirable behavior became more regular than before, and by the end of three months' of school, she was vomiting every day in class. The teacher responded to this practice by sending Laura back to her dormitory, especially when she had vomited on her own clothes. Since this procedure did not stop her behavior problem, Laura eventually was dismissed from class. Tantrums, such as screaming, tearing her clothes, and destroying property also accompanied each of Laura's vomiting episodes in class. Because school was a crucial part of her socialization, elimination of Laura's problems was very important Drug therapy had been employed, but it proved unsuccessful.

Consequently, to reduce Laura's vomiting, an Extinction procedure was attempted. In general, the operations were as follows:

1. From the information that Laura had been returned to her dormitory following her vomiting episodes, the authors guessed that this measure positively reinforced Laura's undesirable behavior and, therefore, perpetuated it.
2. Consequently, two months after Laura had been dismissed from class, she was brought back, but this time Laura's new teacher was instructed not to send her to the dormitory if she vomited. Laura returned only when class was over, regardless of how many times she vomited. In short, what was believed to func-

---

[8]Montrose M. Wolf, Jay S. Birnbrauer, Tom Williams, and Julia Lawler, "A note on apparent extinction of the vomiting behavior of a retarded child," in *Case Studies in Behavior Modification*, eds. L. P. Ullmann and L. Krasner (New York: Holt, Rinehart & Winston, Inc., 1965), pp. 364–366.

tion as the positive reinforcer, being sent back to the dormitory, no longer followed the behavior of regurgitation—the contingency was disrupted.

The results of the procedure after 30 days of class clearly showed that vomiting had decreased to zero. In addition, the tantrums, which had accompanied the vomiting, decelerated during this period. One of the most important results of this Extinction method was that desirable classroom behaviors became accelerated. The authors indicated that the child appeared to take increased interest in her daily activities at school.

It has been suggested that undesirable behaviors can interfere with the performance of desirable ones. Thus, it is much more difficult for the nurse to positively reinforce appropriate conduct if unwanted activity is interfering with it. In this case study, Laura's education in school was limited severely by her undesirable, interfering vomiting and tantrums, and only when these problems were dealt with was she able to learn effectively.

The reader may be curious about why Extinction was used in this case, in contrast to one of the other procedures for decelerating undesirable behavior. No clear explanation is available. Other methods also might have proved successful. In this instance, however, the authors were able to ascertain what was perpetuating the undesirable vomiting, that is, what was functioning as the positive reinforcer; so simply discontinuing this reinforcer was the easiest first approach. If Extinction had not been successful, then either Withdrawal of Positive Reinforcement or Aversive Stimulation or both might have been implemented. A nurse's observation and record of the problem, in addition to her understanding and experience with behavior modification principles, will help in deciding which procedure or combination of methods to apply in each case.

In sum, this case study has shown how Extinction was used to reduce the undesirable behavior of a retarded child. By observing that the child was sent back to the dormitory each time she had vomited in class, the authors were able to guess correctly that this consequence was positively reinforcing the unwanted vomiting. Therefore, they instructed the child's teacher to discontinue providing the positive reinforcer; that is, they instructed the teacher not to send the child back to her dormitory when vomiting occurred. The results indicated that vomiting and the associated tantrum behaviors decreased completely within a month of class. In addition, the child began performing appropriate and adaptive activities, once the undesirable ones had diminished.

Application 13. Extinction of Problem Behavior in a Mental Hospital

To illustrate the use of Extinction procedures in a mental hospital, the first part of an informative study entitled *The Psychiatric Nurse as a Behavioral Engineer* (Ayllon and Michael, 1959)[9] will be presented. This example of Extinction does not represent a serious behavior problem but rather one which did prove intractable to other therapeutic approaches. Extremely disturbing patients' problems (e.g., self-injurious behavior) also are modifiable by using the procedures described in this book; perhaps severe difficulties yield more to the methods mentioned previously and to the ones that will be discussed than to any other treatment approaches.

This case study concerns a female mental patient named Lucille, who very often hampered the nurses' work by coming into their office. This undesirable and bothersome behavior had been occurring for two years. "Because the patient was classified as mentally defective, the nurses had resigned themselves to tolerating her behavior."[10] At times, however, Lucille was told not to come into the office, and she had to be forcibly removed when she disobeyed instructions.

In order to decelerate this bothersome conduct, the nurses employed an Extinction procedure. The first step consisted of ascertaining what event might follow the undesirable behavior and might function as a positive reinforcer. It was believed that attention from the ward nurses, even though at times negative, was taking place after the activity and was perpetuating it. Consequently, to decelerate the undesirable behavior, the nurses stopped all forms of attention when Lucille walked into the office; that is, when Lucille entered the room, the nurses made neither positive nor negative comments to her. They discontinued the positive reinforcer (attention).

The results of Extinction became evident when the authors compared the number of the patient's visits to the office before the program had begun to the number of her visits during it. Before Extinction had started, Lucille would enter the office approximately 16 times a day. By the seventh week of the Extinction plan, Lucille's

---

[9]Teodoro Ayllon and Jack Michael, "The psychiatric nurse as a behavioral engineer," *Journal of the Experimental Analysis of Behavior*, 2, 1959, 323–334. Copyright 1959 by the Society for the Experimental Analysis of Behavior, Inc. Additional information and related research may be found in *The Token Economy: A Motivational System for Therapy and Rehabilitation* by T. Ayllon and N. H. Azrin (New York: Appleton-Century-Crofts, 1968).

[10]Ibid., p. 326.

visits had been reduced to approximately two per day. Thus, when the positive reinforcer (attention), believed to be perpetuating the occurrence of the undesirable behavior, was removed, a reduction in Lucille's activity to a reasonable level resulted.

The authors of this study reported that four other cases were treated with Extinction; in all of them, the positive reinforcer eliminated was attention.

Before the behavior modification procedures were implemented, the nurses had observed and had recorded the patient's problem behaviors. These practices took approximately one to three minutes every half hour, which totaled about forty minutes of a nurse's daily work period. The reduction in bothersome and undesirable patient activities, which inordinately complicated the nurses' work, certainly made the time spent in these aspects of behavior modification worthwhile (see Chapter 5).

TERMS AND QUESTIONS

Terms

Extinction of positively reinforced behavior

Questions

1. Describe how the Extinction procedure disrupts a contingency?
2. Why is it important to be consistent when using an Extinction method?
3. How may you apply Extinction to self-injurious behavior?

4.6 *A COMPARISON OF SOME OF THE DECELERATION PROCEDURES*

Aversive Stimulation and Withdrawal of Positive Reinforcement

Both these procedures involve contingent relationships between behavior and events following it. Aversive Stimulation involves the occurrence of the undesirable behavior followed by the presentation of an unpleasant event, such as a shock, a slap, or a loud no. Withdrawal of Positive Reinforcement involves the occurrence of the undesirable behavior followed by the removal of a pleasant event, such as the opportunity to continue playing or eating or the loss of points accumulating for the purchase of some favored activity or object.

Both are effective in decelerating undesirable behavior. The major distinction between these procedures, besides their procedural differences, has to do with the potential occurrence of undesired side effects (see Section 4.2), which are more likely to be a by-product of the Aversive Stimulation than the Withdrawal of Positive Reinforcement procedure. It is impossible, however, to state definitely that Aversive Stimulation will always be accompanied by these negative side effects; research on this procedure is still taking place.

The most effective strategy with the majority of behavior problems is to combine deceleration methods with Positive Reinforcement; that is, deceleration may be applied to reduce undesirable behavior at the same time that Positive Reinforcement is being implemented to accelerate desirable behavior. This combination will be indispensable if the undesirable behavior is preventing the desirable behavior from occurring. For example, if a child frequently engages in temper tantrums, it will be difficult if not impossible, to teach him academic skills without simultaneously attempting to reduce his undesirable behavior. Also, one way to promote long-lasting deceleration of unwanted behavior is to accelerate wanted behavior that is incompatible with it (see Section 4.7).

Extinction and Aversive Stimulation

Both Extinction and Aversive Stimulation can be used to decelerate behavior, but these procedures are very different from each other. As stated, Aversive Stimulation involves a contingent relationship between the occurrence of the undesirable behavior and the presentation of the distasteful event (i.e., the unwanted activity results in the presentation of the aversive event). Extinction, in contrast, does not involve a contingent relationship between behavior and the happenings following it. Extinction involves the disruption of the contingency (i.e., the behavior is no longer followed by the positive reinforcers that previously followed it).

To illustrate the differences between these two procedures, let us consider how one may decelerate a very deviant behavior prevalent in some psychotic children, namely, head banging, which, if left untreated, may result in the death or disfigurement of a youngster.

Suppose that for some of these children, we can identify *attention* from the hospital staff as the probable positive reinforcer for the deviant behavior. If attention is positively reinforcing this self-destructive activity in a psychotic child, we may decelerate it by discontinuing attention; that is, when the child is banging his head the nurses may ignore him. This method is Extinction.

We also may implement Aversive Stimulation. Each time the child is head banging we may shock him with a prod. In other words, a contingency between head banging and the presentation of shock may be established, which will decelerate this undesirable behavior.

Both these procedures are likely to be successful. But there is evidence (Lovaas and Simmons, 1969) that Aversive Stimulation produces more rapid results than Extinction in decelerating self-destructive behavior. Because such conduct is extremely dangerous to the patient, the quickest procedure, if it does not produce undesirable side effects, is the best one. No definitive evidence exists, however, as to which method is the more effective one for every problem.

But whether Aversive Stimulation or Extinction is employed, each is more effective in producing long-lasting changes if used in conjunction with Positive Reinforcement. Self-destructive behavior, for example, certainly interferes with the child's learning appropriate conduct. When self-destruction is held in check by Aversive Stimulation or by Extinction, however, new activities can be accelerated via Positive Reinforcement; they may be incompatible with self-injurious behavior, resulting in its durable reduction.

Extinction and Withdrawal of Positive Reinforcement

Often, these two procedures are difficult to distinguish since both involve the removal of some positive reinforcer. There are, however, two important differences between them.

The first difference is that Withdrawal of Positive Reinforcement results in the positive reinforcer being removed *only* when the behavior occurs (a contingency). Extinction, on the other hand, results in the positive reinforcer being discontinued and no longer following the occurrence of the behavior (i.e., the previous contingency is disrupted, and no reinforcement is administered after the activity). Therefore, in Withdrawal of Positive Reinforcement, the removal of the positive reinforcer is contingent on the occurrence of the behavior, whereas this relationship is not the case in Extinction.

Suppose, for example, that one of the problems of a particular female mental patient is stealing food (see Ayllon, 1963). More specifically, let us say that she takes food from the diningroom counter as well as from other patients during mealtimes. If the patient is removed from the diningroom only when she attempts to pilfer, and the thievery decreases, a Withdrawal of Positive Reinforcement procedure is operating. Suppose, however, that this patient's behavior is being positively reinforced by attention, then simply ignoring the occurrence of this activity exemplifies the Extinction method; that is, the positive reinforcer (attention) is discontinued and, therefore, no longer is able to reinforce the patient's stealing.

The second difference between Withdrawal of Positive Reinforcement and Extinction has to do with whether the positive reinforcer removed is the one perpetuating the behavior. When Withdrawal of Positive Reinforcement is employed, the positive reinforcer eliminated is not necessarily the one which has been perpetuating the problem. In our example, the patient's presence in the diningroom was not necessarily positively reinforcing her stealing food. But being in the diningroom was a positive reinforcer whose removal (i.e., Withdrawal of Positive Reinforcement) was effective in obliterating the stealing problem. When Extinction is used, the discontinued positive reinforcer is always the one perpetuating the behavior. If the positive reinforcers maintaining the undesirable activity are not known or are difficult to eliminate completely, either the Withdrawal of Positive Reinforcement or Aversive Stimulation procedures should be employed.

QUESTIONS

1. What is the major procedural difference between Aversive Stimulation and Withdrawal of Positive Reinforcement?
2. How do Extinction and Aversive Stimulation differ as procedures?
3. What are the two major differences between Extinction and Withdrawal of Positive Reinforcement?
4. Why should one always try to incorporate Positive Reinforcement in any behavior modification program?

4.7 REINFORCING OTHER BEHAVIOR

Description and Treatment Definition

This approach for decelerating undesirable behavior utilizes the Positive Reinforcement procedure. Positive Reinforcement may be employed *alone* to accelerate desirable behavior, *which can prevent undesirable behavior from occurring.* Using Positive Reinforcement in this way involves *Reinforcing Other Behavior* that is *incompatible* with the activity the nurse wants to reduce or to eliminate.

Consider once again, the example of the mental patient who complained about strange odors on the ward and who, in general, resisted going to bed at night (see Extinction, Section 4.5). If the nurses decided that they would positively reinforce the patient when he was *not* complaining, no matter what else he was doing, the grumbling would decrease soon. In other words, all those activities which did not involve complaining would be more likely to occur than complaining *per se.* Complaining and not complaining are two activities which cannot occur at the same time; consequently, they are incompatible. When the patient is provided with new means of obtaining positive reinforcers other than the undesirable ways, his problems will decrease. In this example, if attention from the nurses were a positive reinforcer for this patient, a nurse may compliment the patient periodically for his good behavior. One very effective way of decreasing an undesirable behavior, therefore, is to accelerate an incompatible activity via the Positive Reinforcement procedure. The treatment definition of Reinforcing Other Behavior is as follows:

Reinforcing Other Behavior is a procedure in which an unwanted activity is decreased by administering positive reinforcers contingent on the occurrence of desirable behavior which is incompatible with the undesirable behavior. An incompatible behavior is any activity that does not occur at the same time as the undesirable behavior.

There are basically two kinds of incompatible behavior that the nurse can accelerate:

1. *Any behavior occurring after time has elapsed in which the undesirable behavior has not occurred.* For instance, if the undesirable behavior was screaming, and if the patient remained quiet for two minutes, he could be given reinforcers at the end

of this two minute period no matter what he was doing, as long as he was not yelling.

2. *Some specific behavior found incompatible with the undesirable behavior.* For example, Lovaas, Freitag, Gold, and Kassorla (1965) positively reinforced a child whenever she made an appropriate response to music in order to reduce her self-destructive behavior; her suitable reactions, such as clapping hands, were incompatible with being self-destructive.

With either of these two kinds of incompatible behavior, the positive reinforcers used may be the same ones which originally perpetuated the undesirable behavior. For example, if attention were positively reinforcing screaming, attention could be made to immediately follow and, thereby, to positively reinforce a period of not screaming. In effect, this would provide the patient with an appropriate alternative way of receiving the same type of reinforcer.

Additional Comments

The use of Positive Reinforcement, an acceleration procedure, to prevent unwanted behavior from occurring is a very effective manipulation. It makes sense that one way to remove an undesirable activity is to develop an incompatible desirable one. If a teacher wishes to stop a child from continually leaving his seat, she may punish him when he gets up from his chair. But she also may positively reinforce him for staying in his seat. Or, as indicated previously and as will be discussed in Section 4.8, she may use both approaches.

Application 14. Reinforcing Other Behavior in a Mental Hospital Patient

This example was abstracted from Allyon and Michael's (1959) article entitled *The Psychiatric Nurse as a Behavioral Engineer,*[11] which was referred to in Section 4.5 (Extinction). Reinforcing Other Behavior was used to decelerate the violent activity of the female patient described below:

> Dotty, had become increasingly violent over the last five years, and recently attacked several patients and hospital personnel without any apparent reason. Since admission and up to the present, she

[11]Ayllon and Michael, op. cit., pp. 323–334.

> had received many electroconvulsive-therapy treatments aimed at reducing this violence, with little or no success. In 1947, a physician recommended her as a good case for psychosurgery. In December of the same year, she attempted to strangle her mother, who was visiting her at the time. In July 1948, the patient had a leucotomy. The situation had recently become so serious that at the least suspicious move on her part the nurses would put her in the seclusion room. She spent from 3 to 12 hours daily in that room.[12]

To reduce this patient's violence by Reinforcing Other Behavior, it was necessary to discover an activity incompatible with her outbursts. In short, the nurses needed to reinforce some response that did not occur at the same time as Dotty's frenzy. It was observed that one of the nonviolent behaviors this patient engaged in was being on the floor ("lying, squatting, kneeling, sitting"). When Dotty was on the floor, she was not violent. Consequently, the nurses administered positive reinforcers to the patient by making socially approving comments to her when she was on the floor. In addition, the nurses positively reinforced Dotty's meaningful approaches toward them; that is, when Dotty made a request or a comment or asked a question, the nurses gave her social approval.

The nurses recorded both the number of times Dotty had been on the floor and the number of desirable approach-responses she had made.

The results showed that the behavior of being on the floor increased, but more important the undesirable violent behavior decreased. In addition, the desirable act of asking the nurse questions, for example, occurred more frequently than before. But when Dotty was no longer reinforced for being on the floor, her outbursts returned. Thus, being on the floor was incompatible with being violent. When being on the floor was positively reinforced, her tumultuous behaviors decreased; when being on the floor was no longer reinforced, these behaviors increased.

This application was presented to show the use of the Reinforcing Other Behavior procedure. By strengthening conduct incompatible with the undesirable activity, the nurses were able to decelerate the undesirable activity temporarily.

Perhaps, a more gradual approach from reinforcing the behavior of being on the floor to reinforcing all of the positive interac-

---

[12]Ibid., pp. 328–329.

tions with the nurses could have been attempted. Intermediate steps between being on the floor and desirably dealing with nurses may have been positively reinforced. These interactions may then have become incompatible with violent behavior. In other words, through the techniques of *Shaping, Demonstration–Imitation, Instructing,* and so on positive dealings with the nurses and even other patients may have been accelerated and may have become inharmonious with the unwanted violent activities. Since these interactions are more likely to be positively reinforced by other patients as well as by the staff than is being on the floor, the reduction in this patient's undesirable behavior may have been more durable.

TERMS AND QUESTIONS

Terms

Incompatible behavior
Reinforcing Other Behavior procedure

Questions

1. How may you use the Reinforcing Other Behavior procedure to reduce the hoarding problem of the patient discussed in Application 11? What may be a major difficulty in applying this procedure to this problem?
2. How may you apply the Reinforcing Other Behavior procedure in Application 13?

4.8 *COMBINING ACCELERATION AND DECELERATION PROCEDURES*

To maximize the effectiveness and the meaningfulness of employing deceleration procedures, it is often advisable to combine one or more of them with Positive Reinforcement; Negative Reinforcement also may be used together with one or more of the deceleration procedures (e.g., Lovaas, Schaeffer, and Simmons, 1965).

Throughout this chapter, it has been suggested that if constructive alternative activities are made available to the patient—if the patient is positively reinforced for desirable behavior that competes with the undesirable behavior—the likelihood of other deviant activities arising (see symptom substitution, Chapter 1) or undesirable side effects occurring is reduced; also, the probability of producing durable change, that is, long-lasting deceleration of undesirable behavior is greater. In many cases, it is possible to alter the reinforcement contingency such that the reinforcer (e.g., attention) that previously followed the deviant behavior is made to follow a desirable set of activities.

When a combination of acceleration and deceleration procedures are used for one patient, the nurse must be careful to properly define both the activities to be accelerated and to be decelerated. The target behaviors to be accelerated should be labeled *Ta,* and the ones to be decelerated should be labeled *Td.* The rules of application discussed for Positive Reinforcement procedure and for each one of the deceleration methods should be followed when acceleration and deceleration operations are combined.

Some frequently used combinations are as follows: *Positive Reinforcement and Aversive Stimulation; Positive Reinforcement and Withdrawal of Positive Reinforcement; Positive Reinforcement and Extinction.* (Other combinations are possible.)

When these combinations are applied, as when the procedures are used separately, it is important to be systematic and consistent. For example, if Positive Reinforcement and Aversive Stimulation are being used to reduce self-slapping in a psychotic child, each occurrence of the this activity (*Td*) must result in the presentation of the aversive stimulus. And each occurrence of the target behaviors to be accelerated, such as sitting quietly or playing appropriately for 30 seconds (both *Ta*'s) must be followed by the administration of the positive reinforcer.

Once the *Td* has been decelerated, and once the *Ta* has been sufficiently accelerated, an intermittent schedule of reinforcement for the *Ta* can be instituted. But the *Td* should be followed *consistently,* not intermittently, by the presentation of the aversive stimulus. In other words, either a variable ratio or a variable interval schedule can be implemented for the desirable behavior that has been accelerated, but *each* reoccurrence of the undesirable behavior should be followed by its appropriate consequence (e.g., presentation of the aversive stimulus, withdrawal of the positive reinforcer, or simply no reinforcer).

It is important to point out that if the wanted activity rarely or never occurs, one of the techniques for producing behavior discussed in Chapter 3 may be employed in conjunction with the deceleration procedures.

Several of the applications and examples discussed in preceding parts of this book have incorporated a combination of approaches, but these combinations, for purposes of exposition, have not been scrutinized. In the next two applications, however, close attention will be given to the manner in which acceleration and deceleration procedures have been used together.

Application 15. Using Positive Reinforcement and Extinction Procedures to Modify the Speech of a Mental Patient

Only the first case study in an article (Ayllon and Haughton, 1964)[13] concerning the inappropriate speech patterns of three female mental patients will be reported. The individual considered here was described by the authors as follows:

> Kathy was a 47-year-old female patient diagnosed as chronic schizophrenic. She had been in the hospital for 16 years. The patient's verbal behavior centered around so-called "delusions." The content of her verbal behavior was characterized by frequent references to "Queen Elizabeth," "King George," and the "Royal Family." A sample of her talk is as follows: "I'm the Queen. Why don't you give things to the Queen? The Queen wants to smoke . . . How's King George, have you seen him?" These self-references were traced through hospital records and had been reported over the preceding 14 years. The staff stated that references to herself as "the Queen" had been virtually her only topic of conversation for the eight years immediately prior to this investigation. . . .[14]

Two types of speech content were selected for behavior modification: The *psychotic type,* which included statements such as those indicated above, and the *neutral type,* which included any statement that was not psychotic (e.g., "What time is it," "I'd like some soap." thus, the target behaviors were neutral statements (*Ta*) and psychotic statements (*Td*).

The statements to be accelerated (*Ta*) were positively reinforced by the nurses; that is, a nurse demonstrated interest in what the patient was saying by sometimes offering her a cigarette or a piece of candy and at other times by "lighting a cigarette herself

---

[13] T. Ayllon and E. Haughton, "Modification of symptomatic verbal behaviour of mental patients," *Behaviour Research and Therapy,* 2, 1964, 87–97.

[14] Ibid., p. 90.

and joining the patient." If the patient made psychotic statements (*Td*), the above-mentioned reinforcers were not given (Extinction). Apparently, this behavior previously had garnered attention and interest from the hospital staff.

Both procedures were carried out in three-minute periods; that is, each verbal interaction between the patient and a nurse was three minutes long. When the patient approached a nurse, the latter attempted to stay with her during this period and to implement either the Positive Reinforcement or the Extinction procedure.

The effectiveness of Positive Reinforcement and Extinction in altering this patient's speech was demonstrated clearly. When psychotic statements *Td*'s) no longer were reinforced (Extinction), they were markedly reduced, and when neutral statements (*Ta*'s) were reinforced positively they were markedly increased. This phase of the study took 90 days and followed a period where, for research purposes, the reverse of the relationships above were in effect.

In sum, the verbal behavior of this mental patient was altered by changing its social consequences. Similar results were obtained with two other patients who evidenced repetitive somatic complaints such as "My nerves are shot" and "I can't hear anymore."

As the authors pointed out, attempts to treat patients, such as the one described, by humoring them or by explaining to them that their statements are incorrect may have deteriorative results. A patient's verbal complaints or psychotic statements can be reinforced by attention from the hospital staff; that is, paying attention to these behaviors can accelerate the problem. *Ignoring these statements* and *attending to appropriate verbalizations,* on the other hand, can have desirable results.

Application 16. Combining Positive Reinforcement and Withdrawal of Positive Reinforcement Via a Behavioral Contract for Losing Weight

Obesity is a problem that bothers many persons. In the present study, (Mann, 1971),[15] this intractable problem was modified by relatively simple measures.

Briefly, Positive Reinforcement for weight loss (*Ta*) and Withdrawal of Positive Reinforcement for weight gain (*Td*) were implemented through a behavioral contract; contracts have been men-

---

[15]Ronald A. Mann, "The use of contingency contracting to control obesity in adult subjects." Paper presented at the meeting of the Western Psychological Association, San Francisco, California, 1971.

tioned previously (see Chapter 3, Section 3.2). The nine adults who participated in this study and who volunteered because they complained of being overweight helped to stipulate the clauses.

Each behavioral contract specified the various ways in which the participant could earn and could lose reinforcers—valuable items, such as money and jewelry, which each overweight person had given to the author before the contract went into effect. Specifically, the agreement required the following:

1. That each adult be weighed regularly by the author.
2. That each adult specify the minimum amount he expected to lose every two weeks.
3. That each adult specify the amount he expected to weigh by the end of the program (his terminal weight).

Therefore, the contract was tailored to each individual.

As stipulated, participants regained or forfeited reinforcers in the following ways:

1. Each time an adult lost two pounds, the author returned one of his valuables (Positive Reinforcement procedure). But each time he gained two pounds, he forfeited permanently one of his valuables to the author (Withdrawal of Positive Reinforcement procedure). The participants were weighed regularly.
2. Because each adult had specified how much he had expected to lose every two weeks, he was weighed at the end of each two-week period. One valuable was given if the stipulated weight reduction requirement was fulfilled (Positive Reinforcement). But if he did not meet this condition, a participant forfeited that valuable (Withdrawal of Positive Reinforcement).
3. The same contingencies operated for the terminal weight requirement; that is, if the adult attained his stipulated goal by the end of the program, he received several valuables, which had been set aside in the contract for this purpose and, therefore, never were in jeopardy of being lost or capable of being won during the plan. In addition, the contract stipulated that all remaining valuables (i.e., those neither won nor lost) be given to the adult once he reached his goal. If anyone quit the program, however, he forfeited all these esteemed personal possessions. They became the property of the author. (Because he wanted to estimate the effectiveness of his procedures, the au-

thor reserved the right to implement evaluative techniques, which will be discussed in the next chapter.)

After all these arrangements were written down to form a contract, the participants signed it. The contract, therefore, clearly and definitively stated how positive reinforcers could be regained or forfeited. Special reinforcers were unnecessary; that is, all the reinforcers incorporated into the program were already available to each adult and, according to the statements of each, were potent. In other words, the items used to modify obesity were available in the setting in which the behavior modification program was carried out and did not have to be arbitrarily imposed by the investigator. The contract simply helped to arrange contingencies between target behaviors (i.e., losing weight, gaining weight) and reinforcers.

The results indicated that these simple manipulations were effective. Five of the participants reached their terminal goal; that is, they were 100% successful by the end of the program. One adult was 70% successful, and the three other individuals ranged between being 40% and 52% successful. Thus, all the participants lost weight. One, in fact, lost 102 pounds.

In sum, overweight adults, who were essentially healthy in other respects, were helped through a system of contingent Positive Reinforcement and contingent Withdrawal of Positive Reinforcement. Each participant surrendered specific items he considered valuable to the author. They served as reinforcers and were used to accelerate weight loss (*Ta*) and to decelerate weight gain (*Td*). Both Positive Reinforcement and Withdrawal of Positive Reinforcement were implemented via a tailored behavioral contract that explicitly and carefully delineated the ways in which each adult could regain or could lose reinforcers. According to the results, combining Positive Reinforcement and Withdrawal of Positive Reinforcement in the framework of a written agreement was highly effective.

This strategy is applicable to various behavior problems that the nurse encounters, particularly in natural settings with noninstitutionalized adults and children.

TERMS AND QUESTIONS

Terms

Ta

Td

Questions

1. What are the advantages of combining acceleration and deceleration procedures in one behavior modification program?
2. What must be done in order to implement effectively a combination of acceleration and deceleration procedures? Be brief.
3. How would you combine Positive Reinforcement and Withdrawal of Positive Reinforcement in Application 12?
4. Using Positive Reinforcement and any deceleration procedure, how will you reduce the disobedience of a 10-year-old well child?
5. Using a combination of methods, how can you help a child who is chronically constipated? Assume that no medical reason exists for his condition (a variety of medical remedies have already been tried but have not been durable).

4.9 *A SYNTHESIS*

This chapter has dealt with five procedures for decelerating behavior. Three of them (Aversive Stimulation, Withdrawal of Positive Reinforcement, Reinforcing Other Behavior), involve contingent relationships between the occurrence of behavior and the presentation or removal of some consequence; Reinforcing Other Behavior is the Positive Reinforcement procedure applied to accelerate an activity incompatible with the behavior to be decelerated. The two remaining methods (Extinction and Satiation) do *not* involve contingent relationships; that is, neither the contingent presentation nor the contingent removal of a particular consequence results from the occurrence of the undesirable behavior. Extinction, for instance, involves the disruption of the contingency between an activity and its consequences (i.e., positive reinforcers are simply discontinued).

The deceleration procedures must be applied consistently. For example, if Aversive Stimulation is being implemented, each occurrence of the undesirable behavior should be followed by the presentation of the distasteful agent. Or, if Withdrawal of Positive Reinforcement is being used, each occurrence of the target behavior should result in the removal of some positive reinforcer. Or, if Extinction is being employed, no occurrences of the undesirable target behavior should be followed by the positive reinforcer. In short, a continuous application of consequences is more effective than an intermittent one. The specific rules and comments pertinent to applying each of the deceleration procedures were given in this chapter.

As yet, it is impossible to state definitively which of the deceleration procedures is most appropriate in any one case. The least physically painful methods (e.g., Withdrawal of Positive Reinforcement, Extinction), however, have the added advantage of not being so strongly associated with undesirable side effects. But Aversive Stimulation may be a more potent procedure for rapidly decelerating extremely dangerous behavior (e.g., self-destruction). With less injurious behavior, such as crying or hyperactivity, Extinction or Withdrawal of Positive Reinforcement both seem to be effective and may be tried initially. And with still other types of problems (e.g., hoarding), Satiation has been shown to be useful.

Careful and continual monitoring of the fluctuations in the patient's behaviors is the best guide to changing procedures which are not serving in his best interests. In addition, the experience and good judgment of the nurse-practitioner are indispensable both for effectively implementing the methods and for altering them after the program has begun.

Long lasting behavior changes are more likely to occur if the deceleration approaches are combined with the Positive Reinforcement procedure. The potential occurrences of undesirable side effects and the development of new undesirable behaviors are less likely, and the transient effects that can be found in behavior modification programs are less probable if Positive Reinforcement is applied to constructive behavior. A combination of acceleration and deceleration procedures is more likely to result in durable behavior changes—changes which last after the behavior modification program has ended—than no such combination.

To modify undesirable behavior, it is valuable to accelerate desirable activities that compete with the occurrence of undesirable ones. Thus, administering reinforcers to a retarded child for diligently working at his desk on some task in conjunction with withdrawing reinforcers when he is noisy (e.g., placing him in Time-Out) or ignoring his noisy behaviors (e.g., Extinction) are effective combinations for reducing the child's undesirable conduct. With this approach, the same reinforcers that the child obtained for being noisy, such as *attention from the teacher,* can be reprogrammed to follow the behavior of working diligently. In this way, the child will be helped to obtain the same potent positive reinforcers by performing constructive activities rather than by engaging in unwanted ones. Similar statements may be made for many people with different behavior problems. Simply stated, deceleration procedures are likely to be most effective, when the Positive Reinforcement procedure is also incorporated into the behavior change program.

Relatedly, if the nurse's goal is to accelerate the desirable behaviors of the patient, Positive Reinforcement will be facilitated if the undesirable behaviors that compete with this goal also are decelerated. Thus, helping a mental hospital patient to participate actively in ward meetings by positively reinforcing his appropriate comments is more likely to be successful if the patient's frequent inattendance or his abrupt departure from the meetings are fined; the penalty may consist of the removal of tokens on a token-economy ward, or it may consist of the loss of some privilege. Desirable behavior should payoff, and undesirable behavior should cost.

A behavioral contract is one method whereby acceleration and deceleration procedures can be productively combined (Homme et al., 1971). This strategy is useful in many situations (e.g., school and home) and for various problems (e.g., delinquency, truancy, and obesity). Behavioral contracts clearly and definitively spell out the contingencies. Each participant knows *what* behavior in *each* situation will be followed by *which* consequence. Thus, there is openness and fairness in the agreement. Each participant knows what is expected of him and what to expect from others. Furthermore, because all parties must agree about the clauses in the contract, control over behavior is granted, not appropriated. This approach to modifying behavior seems especially relevant to the pursuits of nurses involved in the schools and in the community.

Both Chapters 3 and 4 have elucidated the procedures for altering behavior. In the next chapter, the activities of the nurse essential for assessment and evaluation will be discussed.

SUPPLEMENTARY READINGS

BAER, D. M. "A Case for the Selective Reinforcement of Punishment," in *Behavior Modification in Clinical Psychology,* eds. C. Neuringer and J. L. Michael. New York: Appleton-Century-Crofts, 1970.

BANDURA, A. *Principles of Behavior Modification.* New York: Holt, Rinehart & Winston, Inc., 1969, pp. 308–313.

BLACKHAM, G. J., AND A. SILBERMAN *Modification of Child Behavior.* Belmont, California: Wadsworth Publishing Company, Inc., 1971, pp. 78–91.

LOVAAS, O. I., G. FREITAG, VIVIAN J. GOLD, AND IRENE C. KASSORLA "Experimental Studies in Childhood Schizophrenia: Analysis of Self-Destructive Behavior," *Journal of Experimental Child Psychology,* 2, 1965, 67–84.

LOVAAS, O. I., AND J. Q. SIMMONS "Manipulation of Self-Destruction in Three Retarded Children," *Journal of Applied Behavior Analysis,* 2, 1969, 143–157.

RESNICK, J. H. "The Control of Smoking Behaviour by Stimulus Satiation," *Behaviour Research and Therapy,* 6, 1968, 113–114.

WALTON, D. "The Application of Learning Theory to the Treatment of a Case of Neurodermatitis," in *Behaviour Therapy and the Neuroses,* ed. H. J. Eysenck. London: Pergamon Press, 1960.

WOLF, M. M., T. RISLEY, AND H. MEES "Application of Operant Conditioning Procedures to the Behaviour Problems of an Autistic Child," *Behaviour Research and Therapy,* 1, 1964, 305–312.

five | *Designing and Evaluating Behavior Modification Programs*

5.1 *INTRODUCTORY COMMENTS AND THE IMPORTANCE OF ACCURATE DEFINITIONS*

To successfully carry out a behavior modification program for an individual, the nurse-practitioner must be accurate, precise, and critical about what she is doing. These overlapping adjectives describe the nurse who skillfully designs, implements, and evaluates a plan. Imprecise or haphazard approaches to changing behavior are likely to have either no positive effects or, worse, negative ones; that is, the patient's behaviors deteriorate.

As indicated in Chapter 1, a behavior modification program proceeds through three stages: *Assessment* of the problems; *Intervention* to remedy the problems (i.e., either by accelerating certain behaviors, by decelerating certain behaviors, or by a combination); *Evaluation* to ascertain if the intervention techniques are working correctly and if they have caused the changes that have occurred. These stages are related to one another in ways which this chapter will indicate.

Thus far, we have discussed the basic Intervention procedures (e.g., Positive Reinforcement and Extinction). The focus of this chapter, however, is on Assessment, Evaluation and the necessary qualities of the nurse who carries out these activities. The three important components of assessing a patient's behavior are defining it, observing it, and recording it; this section will be concerned with the first element, namely, defining behavior.

Accurately Defining the Patient's Behavior So That It Can Be Observed and Recorded

In order to observe and to record precisely a patient's behavior, both desirable and undesirable, it is first necessary to define it accurately.

Often we describe behavior in very general and nonspecific ways. For instance we say that Mr. *Q.* is schizophrenic, or Miss *R.* is unhappy, or Johnny is passive, or Mrs. *P* is angry, or Mr. *Z* is aggressive. These types of global description are not really very useful for the behavior modifier. What does it mean to say that Mr. Z is aggressive? Does it mean that he strikes nurses when he is in the hospital? Does it mean that he speaks up when he feels he should, no matter where he is? Does it mean that he makes threats? Does it mean that he is a Don Juan who is outspoken with the ladies? Or does it mean all of these descriptions, several of these, one of these, or even none of these? The point is that to understand the word *aggressive* it has to be defined objectively. For behavior modification, the terms used to depict a person's behavior have to be defined in such a way that what is meant can be observed and recorded.

An accurate definition of a patient's behavior, therefore, incorporates specific statements about what he does or does not do. More precisely, the definition of Mr. *Z*'s behavior must be accurate and clear enough for at least two separate observers to agree that the behavior occurred or did not occur. This stipulation is the *observer agreement requirement*; the degree of agreement between observers can be computed (see Section 5.3).

To say that Mr. *Z* "strikes" nurses and "shoves" other patients is more specific than saying that he is "aggressive." But the terms *strike* and *shove* also are somewhat ambiguous. For instance, what constitutes "striking" as opposed to "patting," or "shoving" in contrast to "nudging"? Two separate observers must agree on the definition of a "strike" and the definition of a "shove." Striking another individual may be defined more accurately as any occurrence of Mr. *Z.* swinging his arm or his leg in the direction of another individual, resulting in his making contact with the individual. Some behaviors are easier to define than others, but all activities to be observed precisely and to be recorded must be defined accurately enough to satisfy the observer-agreement requirement.

In the behavior modification literature, many reports of accurate and specific behavioral definitions can be found. For example, O'Leary, O'Leary, and Becker (1967) were able to observe and to record several classes of conduct (e.g., isolate, deviant, and cooperative) for two brothers by accurately defining each class of behavior. Cooperative behavior was explained as asking for a toy, requesting help, conversing, and playing within three feet of one another.

LeBow, Gelfand and Dobson (1970) were able to record the frequency of a mental patient's respiratory strider by defining it as a harsh, high-pitched, inspiratory sound.

Wahler (1969) dealt with oppositional and with cooperative behavior in "oppositional" children. The activities were defined in terms of the youngster's response to parental requests. Briefly, if he complied with his parent's instruction (e.g., "stop jumping on the couch" or "please take out the garbage") for a full ten seconds, his response was recorded as cooperative. If the child did not acquiesce to the request during any portion of the ten-second interval, the behavior was considered oppositional.

The nurses described in Application 15 recorded their conversations with a female mental patient. Psychotic statements were defined as those including references to the "Queen," to the "King," and so on, whereas neutral verbalizations included such utterances as, "It's nice today," or "What time is it?"

From what has been said, it should be clear that accurate definitions of behavior reflect more of what is actually taking place than what the observer infers is occurring. Inferences about behavior, particularly *inferences pertaining to feelings and to motives, cloud a behavioral definition.* This confusion reduces the degree of agreement between observers. Thus, rather than to say that one patient is "angry" at another during their conversation, which you observe, it is more useful to record what each patient does in the situation, that is, the behaviors of each patient. If an individual reports that he's angry, however, this information may be useful for the nurse in designing a behavior modification program. The point is that unconfirmed inferences about internal states, such as saying that a patient is angry because he looks angry, should be avoided.

Preliminary Observations of Behavior Problems

The initial indication that behavior modification is needed is usually some vague statement that there is a problem with a particular person's behavior. Thus, a person is depicted as unhappy, withdrawn, slow to learn, unfriendly, or aggressive, and so forth. Descriptions such as these can be given by the person himself, his family, his friends, his physician, the ward nurse or by several of these individuals. Regardless of who complains first, the early statements made about the problems of an individual, generally, are vague.

The first step in helping any individual, as stated, is to find out what activities are or are not taking place; that is, the first step is to accurately define the problem. Making *preliminary observations* is one approach.

Preliminary observations can be carried out by completely recording a miniature segment of the patient's behavior (Bijou, Peterson, and Ault, 1968). For instance, a nurse may select four 15-minute periods from each day for several days to set down a running description of a patient's activities when he is alone and when he is interacting with others. This recording should take place in the setting where the problems are likely to occur (e.g., the hospital, or the home).

After each behavioral episode is noted, it may be divided into three categories: the behavior—the middle category; the events immediately preceding the behavior—the first category; and the events immediately following the behavior—the last category (Bijou, Peterson and Ault, 1968).

This type of analysis will help the nurse to define events that seem to set the occasion for behavior (antecedents) and events that seem to reinforce it (consequences). From this analysis, accurate definitions can be formulated that later can be observed and recorded *more* precisely. The nurse can observe behaviors, or she can teach others (e.g., teachers, parents, foster grandparents) to gather important information.

Other approaches to formulating definitions are possible. Preliminary observations can be supplemented by interviewing the patient, his family, his physician, or his friends. The interview is useful for gathering information about the patient's problems (i.e., his excesses and his deficits in behavior), the desirable activities he engages in, the potential positive reinforcers that can be employed to change his behavior, as well as the antecedent and consequent situations that control his behavior. If other helping agents will be employed, the initial interview also provides a good time to explain the rationale of behavior modification to them.

TERMS AND QUESTIONS

Terms

Preliminary observation
Observer-agreement requirement

Questions

1. Assessment is the first stage of a behavior modification program. What are the essential parts of assessment, and what are the other two stages of a behavior modification program?
2. Why is it important to define behavior accurately?
3. What constitutes an accurate definition of behavior?
4. What accurate definitions can you make up for these descriptive statements?
   (a) John is aggressive.
   (b) John lacks self-esteem.
   (c) John is apathetic.
5. How can preliminary observations be used to formulate accurate definitions of a patient's behavior? Describe.

5.2 *PRECISELY OBSERVING AND RECORDING BEHAVIOR*

Observing and Recording Behavior as Well as the Events Affecting It

The central event in behavior modification is behavior. Whether an excess or a deficit in a particular behavior is defined as the problem, its frequency must be recorded. The frequency of a behavior is its most useful measurement. But others are possible. For example, duration of behavior (how many seconds or minutes long it lasts) can be employed to gauge the strength of various activities (e.g., how long a child talks to his peers or how long a mental patient attends to a task).

Although in the modification program the patient's behavior is the major event, it is not the only one that the careful nurse observes. *Behavior does not occur in a vacuum.* The activities of other people, in particular, affect our behavior and vice versa. Therefore, it is important to observe and to record the activities of other people that affect the behavior of the patient. *This area includes the activities of other people that may be setting the occasion for the patient's behavior and the activities of other people that may be reinforcing those of the patient.* Thus, if Johnny, a retarded child, has many temper tantrums, the frequency of this behavior should be recorded. In addition, an attempt should be made to find out the events that usually precede it (i.e., the incidents that may be setting the occasion for the behavior) and the events that usually follow it (i.e., the consequences that may be reinforcing the behavior).

It may be observed that Johnny's temper tantrums usually occur during the afternoon in the recreation area when several other children are present. In addition, it may be observed rather consistently that immediately following the onset of Johnny's fit, the nurses attempt to console him, and the other children stare at him. These consequent events may be affecting the activity, and changing them may reduce Johnny's problem. Attention from the nurses and from the other youngsters, for instance, may be presented contingent on Johnny's playing (Positive Reinforcement) and may be removed contingent on his tantrum (Withdrawal of Positive Reinforcement). Thus, by changing the consequences of Johnny's undesirable behavior, the nurses would be able to decelerate it.

It is possible, also, to modify behavior by changing the events that set the occasion for it. For example, a child disobedient in school may be reacting to the incompetent behaviors of his teacher, that is, the teacher's activities may be setting the occasion for the child's misconduct. If this is the case, remedying the teacher's behaviors should become a major objective of the behavior modification program.

The more information we have concerning the behavior of an individual the more likely we will choose appropriate procedures for changing it in a desirable direction. For example, suppose a school nurse is besieged by the continual visits of an overweight seventh grader named Fred. The child visits the nurse's office each day, soon after the one o'clock bell rings, and he stays for about an hour; usually, he complains of nausea.

Several questions are important to ask before intervention is attempted. First, is there any medical reason for Fred's complaint of nausea? Second, if it has no medical basis, what are the other conditions that may be setting the occasion for his visits? Third, what are the possible reinforcers maintaining Fred's visits? Fourth, what behaviors, in addition to his arrivals, do we want to alter?

The frequency of Fred's visits is one per day (in the afternoon). By recording how often he stops by the nurse's office as well as the time he generally comes, we suspect that he is cutting his gym periods; that is, immediately before Fred's arrival at the nurse's office, the one o'clock bell rings signaling gym for all the boys in his grade. Because the bell almost consistently precedes Fred's visits, it is quite likely that he is cutting gym. Through interviews with Fred and with other students and through increased observation, we learn that Fred's gym periods involve competitive activities and that Fred is a poor athlete. In addition, we learn that success at these activities is generously praised by the coaches as well as by the other students but, unfortunately, failure is heavily ridiculed (Aversive Stimulation). And little or no shaping of good performance takes place.

By possessing all this information, the nurse will be able to select several target behaviors that can be altered either separately or together. Thus, one target may involve Fred's weight, and a related one may deal with his athletic abilities. If Fred could lose weight and could become a better athlete, his frequent visits to the nurse probably would decrease; that is, he no longer would avoid gym. The complex events affecting Fred's continuous visits are, among other things, the positive reinforcers (the friendliness and the understanding of the nurse) that he encounters at the office and the ridicule during gym that he is avoiding (Negative Reinforcement) by going to the nurse's office. If the friendliness of the nurse may be made contingent on weight loss and if praise by the coaches may be made contingent on increasing athletic skill (Shaping), Fred's problem behaviors may be resolved.

The point is that the more complete the information concerning an individual's problem behaviors and the events associated with them, the more equipped the nurse will be to design an effective and meaningful intervention plan. In this regard, it is useful to find out about the desirable activities the individual engages in and the events affecting them as well as the potential positive reinforcers that can be employed for change.

Assessing the Target Behavior Before Intervention: Baseline Information

Before behavior modification procedures are implemented, the nurse should observe the target behavior until definitive information on its current frequency is recorded. This information allows her not only to assess precisely the frequency of the target behavior but also to evaluate the effects of the behavior modification procedures on it, once treatment procedures are instituted; that is, knowledge of the frequency of the target behavior before treatment provides the nurse with a base against which to compare the effects of treatment. This observation period, which immediately precedes the implementation of behavior modification procedures, is called *baseline.*

More specifically, a record of activity that gives a precise account of the frequency of the target behavior before any treatment methods are implemented is a *baseline record.* It can be acquired in several weeks of daily observation, in a few hours spread over a day or two, or in other amounts of time. The amount of initial observation necessary varies from one case to another or with the different behaviors of one patient.

The length of the baseline period, however, depends on the fluctuations in the target behavior. Optimally, baseline information should be gathered until the frequency of the activity does not vary much from one observation period to another—until a *stable baseline* is evidenced. A stable baseline is one in which the day-to-day changes in behavior are not excessive. To say that a baseline record is stable involves a judgment by the nurse.

A stable baseline provides the nurse with much information concerning the patient's behavior. These data are useful for monitoring the changes taking place during treatment; that is, by knowing the frequency of the target behavior before treatment, the nurse can evaluate exactly what is occurring during treatment. In addition, this information is useful for evaluating whether the behavior modification procedures per se are responsible for the patient's eventual improvement (see Section 5.4).

If—after one or two weeks of gathering a baseline record of the target behavior—the nurse does not find stability, the behavior modification procedures can still be implemented. In this case, the nurse will have less information with which to evaluate accurately what is taking place, but the practical requirements of the situation may demand the sacrifice. When possible, however, baseline information should be gathered until the baseline record is stable.

To illustrate the difficulty of evaluating what is happening to the target behavior during treatment when the baseline record is unstable, consider the following example. Billy, the patient, hits other children regularly during school hours. If he is observed and the frequency of his aggression is recorded, the data may be as shown in Table 1.

The number of hits on the first day totaled 300; on the second day, 150; on the third day, 50. If behavior modification began on the fourth day (e.g., Withdrawal of Positive Reinforcement), it would be difficult to evaluate whether this procedure was responsible for any further deceleration of the behavior because it was decreasing anyway. Perhaps additional periods of observation over more days would have revealed more stability in the frequency of Billy's hitting, and the effects of a deceleration method on his behavior, therefore, would be more readily apparent.

A stable baseline is one in which no marked *ascending* or *descending* trends in the target behavior are evident, in addition to one in which the fluctuations in the target behavior are not excessive. If a baseline record is descending, as in the above example, or ascending, the application of behavior modification procedures will be difficult to evaluate unless they are implemented to *reverse* the trend (Hall, 1970). Thus, if an autistic child's face slapping is increasing each day, a deceleration procedure aimed at reducing this activity may be applied. Or, conversely, if a mental patient's coherent speech is decreasing each day, a Positive Reinforcement approach designed to accelerate coherent speech may be used.

Regardless of how long a particular person is observed, the

TABLE 1

Observations on the Frequency of One Child's Hitting Other Children During School Hours*

Day No.	*Occurrences Observed Morning (10:00 A.M.)*	*Occurrences Observed Afternoon (1:00 P.M.)*	*Total*
1	160	140	300
2	80	70	150
3	20	30	50

*Fictitious data.

specific *occasions* for observation (e.g., the morning or the evening) should be fixed. Thus, observation may be necessary several times during one day; the times should be decided upon before any observations are carried out and should be used during the baseline and the treatment phases of a behavior modification program (Blackham and Silberman, 1971).

It is also important to specify carefully the particular *settings* in which observations are to be carried out (e.g., the kitchen of the home or the dormitory of the psychiatric ward). If the frequency of some target behavior varies noticeably from one environment to another, this information is significant for designing an intervention plan. Suppose, for instance, that the undesirable behavior (the yelling) of a ten-year-old child occurs four times during three hours in the evening while the child is at home. But at school, in the morning, the behavior occurs thirty times an hour, and in the afternoon at school, it occurs ten times an hour. The differences in these periods and these settings (i.e., home vs. school) are reflected in drastic changes in the frequency of the target behavior. An important question, answerable through more observation, concerns the kinds of events occurring during each of the periods and in each of the settings and their effects on the target behavior. The particular setting in which behavior modification procedures eventually are implemented may depend on this information. Thus, in this example, to treat yelling *only* during the evening, while the child is home, is unwise.

Often baseline records of behavior are not gathered, or the time spent in this activity is too short. Sometimes the problem is very severe, and spending time gathering a baseline record appears inhumane. Arguments for and against obtaining baseline records of behavior can be put forth that will fill many pages of this text. Similar arguments can be put forth about critically evaluating a behavior modification program. The practitioner of change, in the last analysis, has to decide whether the activities mentioned above are important for the patient. In this writer's thinking, the strategy that gives the practitioner the most information about the patient and about his problem is the plan in the best interests of the patient.

In sum, assessing behavior is a vital activity that should be part of every behavior modification project. After they have been defined, the target behaviors to be altered should be observed and should be recorded throughout the behavior modification program. Observations and recordings are made before the behavior change procedures are applied to the target behaviors (baseline), while these methods are being applied (during intervention), and after they have been applied (after intervention). Continual observation and recording yields much information. During intervention, in particular, careful notice of the target behaviors will allow the nurse to alter the behavior modification procedures as necessary; that is, by monitoring the effects of the methods on the target behaviors, the nurse can make sure that the procedures working in the patient's best interests can continue to be used, and those that are not can be altered. The frequent observation of behavior gives the nurse increased control over treatment.

TERMS AND QUESTIONS

Terms

Baseline record
Ascending baseline
Descending baseline
Stable baseline

Questions

1. What should be observed, and what should be recorded?
2. Why is accurate and precise observation so important for an effective behavior modification program?
3. For how long, optimally, should baseline information be gathered?

5.3 *SOME TECHNIQUES FOR PRECISELY RECORDING, CLEARLY SUMMARIZING, AND CORRECTLY EVALUATING OBSERVATIONS OF BEHAVIOR*

Techniques for Precisely Recording Observations

Various ways to record behavior are available (see Hall, 1970). What follows is a brief discussion of three useful techniques. Each is modifiable in accordance with the requirements of the particular case. One other approach—preliminary observation—which involves the continuous recording of everything that occurs, already has been discussed; this technique, as stated, is useful for defining behavior problems.

RECORDING THE FREQUENCY OF ACTIVITIES AS THEY OCCUR. This recording technique is very simple. Specific behaviors, such as the number of times a child asks a question or approaches another youngster in order to play or the frequency with which a hospitalized mental patient refuses requests made by the nurse, can be tallied *as these events occur* and then can be totaled.

Several behaviors can be recorded at one time by making particular symbols, such as *X*, *Y*, or *F*, stand for the particular activities. Each time an act occurs the symbol can be written down on a checklist. Or a running total of the times a behavior takes place can be kept with a wrist counter. (It is available in most sporting goods stores.) A convenient recording method[1] involves placing a number of beans in one pocket and to transferring one bean to another pocket each time the specified behavior occurs; later in the day the total may be computed.

Recording the frequency of a behavior when it occurs does not require the observer to interrupt his activities much (Hall, 1970). All that is needed is for him to press a counter, to jot down a tally mark on a checklist, or to transfer a bean from one pocket to another as soon as the behavior occurs. Because of this advantage, nurses engaged in teaching will find this technique valuable.

RECORDING THE FREQUENCY OF BEHAVIORS IN SPECIFIC INTERVALS (INTERVAL RECORDING). This technique is more elaborate than the previous one, but it yields more information; that is, it gives an indication of both the duration and the frequency of a behavior (Hall, 1970).

For example, suppose you want to know how often a certain paraplegic patient can sustain exercising during ten-minute periods that occur three times a day for him. We may observe him during each of these spans. To increase the accuracy, we may divide each one into small intervals. Therefore, let us divide each ten-minute observation period into 120 five-second intervals (there are 120 five-second spans in ten minutes). Instead of noting his exercising behav-

---

[1]This method was suggested to the author by Donald P. Hartmann, Associate Professor of Psychology at the University of Utah.

ior in ten-minute periods, we will observe it in five-second ones—in 120 five-second intervals.

In each five-second block, we can record whether the patient is exercising (*E*) or whether he has interrupted this activity (*I*). Before we can write down this information, however, we must state some requirement for registering an *E* or an *I*. Let us say that, for our purposes, an *E* (exercise) is recorded if the patient is exercising for at least four seconds during the five-second interval. Thus, if he momentarily stops exercising, an *E* is still scored. Only if he stops for more than one second will an interruption (*I*) be recorded. (We have information, let us suppose, that frequent interruptions retard the physical-therapy program and, therefore, are detrimental to the patient's welfare.)

In this way, armed with watches, an observation form, a clipboard and a pencil, we can record accurately and precisely the frequency of the patient's interruptions (*I*) and his sustained exercising (*E*) during each of the five-second intervals constituting the ten-minute observation period.

Only one score (*E* or *I*) is written down for each five-second block. The objective of this procedure is to ascertain the number of five-second intervals in which sustained exercising occurs.

A sample observation form with fictitious data is presented in Figure 1. For clarity, the form depicts only a total of two minutes, that is, 24 five-second intervals. Twenty-four numbered intervals of five-seconds each (the length of each duration is five seconds) are shown. In each of these spans, either an *E* or an *I* is recorded. It is evident, from the total number of *E*'s, that the patient sustained his exercising during approximately 58% of the intervals, that is, during 14 out of the 24 five-second intervals. Conversely, the patient interrupted his exercising approximately 42% of the time, that is, during 10 out of the 24 five-second intervals. The *stage* of observation is baseline. The *period* of observation is two, but it could have been one or three; there are three observation periods in this hypothetical case.

Interval recording yields much information, but it does require practice and a concerted effort on the part of the observer. During the observation period, his complete and undivided attention must be on his task.

Interval recording can be expanded to incorporate more than one behavior. By adding other columns and by using other symbols, an observer can record the occurrence or nonoccurrence of several activities.

Figure 1

Illustration of an interval-recording form depicting the frequency of sustained exercising for a 30-year-old patient as set down by one nurse.

Name and Age of Patient:	John O., 30 years old
Date of Observation:	September 2
Stage of Observation:	Baseline
Period and Time of Observation:	2 at 2:00 p.m.
Behavior Observed:	Exercising
Number of Intervals Observed:	24
Length of Each Interval:	5 seconds
Total Time of Observation:	2 minutes

Interval Number	Interval Score (Nurse A)
1	E*
2	E
3	E
4	I**
5	E
6	E
7	E
8	I
9	I
10	E
11	I
12	E
13	E
14	I
15	I
16	E
17	I
18	I
19	E
20	E
21	E
22	E
23	I
24	I

* E = an interval wherein exercising was sustained for at least four seconds.

** I = an interval wherein exercising was interrupted for more than one second (exercising was not sustained for at least four seconds).

(All data are fictitious.)

The length of the interval, that is, whether five, two, or forty seconds is used, depends on the frequency of the behavior. *Very frequent* activities require *short* intervals (e.g., five seconds), whereas less frequent activities can be observed in longer spans (e.g., five minutes). If the behavior is relatively infrequent, it can be recorded by other methods, such as by the one mentioned in Item 1.

Variations of the interval-recording method are possible. One of these, which is particularly useful, is to allow the observer a specific amount of time during each interval to stop watching the behavior. During this time, he can write down his observations or rest. For example, he can note the behavior for 10 seconds out of each 15-second interval or for 20 seconds out of each 30-second interval. With this variation, therefore, the observer no longer needs to continuously watch the behavior.

RECORDING THE FREQUENCY OF BEHAVIORS AT THE END OF SPECIFIC INTERVALS (TIME SAMPLING). Although similar to interval recording, time sampling involves one crucial difference. With time sampling, behavior is not observed and is not recorded throughout the interval, but, instead, it is written down *at the end* of the duration (Hall, 1970). For example, with interval recording, the paraplegic patient mentioned above was observed continuously for five seconds before the *I* or the *E* was recorded. If the time-sampling technique had been employed, the patient would have been watched at the end of the five-second interval to see if he was exercising or not. At the end of the designated block, the observer would record whether the patient was performing the specified behavior; this recording would take only a moment to complete.

To some extent, time sampling combines the convenience of the first method discussed, that is, recording the frequency of behavior as it occurs, with the thoroughness of interval recording. Time sampling is applicable to most nursing situations where one or more behaviors need to be observed and recorded.

Schaefer et al. (1966), for example, reported their use of time sampling to record the behavior of mental patients (see Chapter 1). Nurses in the hospital observed specific patients once every half-hour for the occurrence or the nonoccurrence of various behaviors. (e.g., walking, running, standing, sitting, lying down, drinking, eating, pacing, rocking, and chattering); a total of 30 observations per day were made about each patient. These behaviors and others were listed on a form. Each behavior had a number associated with it. Thus, a particular combination of numbers indicated that the patient was engaging in a particular combination of behaviors at the time she was observed (e.g., sitting while rocking and chattering). In addition, the possible locations wherein observations occurred (e.g., bathroom, dining area, sleeping quarters) were coded with different letters.

With this technique, an accurate account of a patient's behavior could be recorded in about one second. By the end of the day, a relatively complete picture of any patient's activities could be obtained. Observations were carried out for several days, and, as mentioned, this information was used for treating "apathy."

There are various ways to construct time sampling observation forms. The form for interval recording may easily be adapted to include several behaviors and the situations wherein these activities occur. In fact, this form may be tailored to fit any individual patient by listing specific behaviors, both desirable and undesirable, particularly important to observe and to record.

The length of the observation interval depends on what you expect to be the frequency of the particular behavior you are going to observe; the size of the interval can be adjusted to fit the purposes of a particular case. Thus, how often a retarded child pays attention to his task can be recorded by observing his behavior once every two minutes; that is, every two minutes in a 30-minute period, the child's teacher can record whether he is looking at the particular materials on his desk or whether he is engaged in other activities. Four of these 30-minute intervals may be arranged for different tasks at varying times of the day.

A sample observation form based on one developed by Schaefer et al. (1969) is shown in Figure 2. The name and age of the patient, the date of the observation, and the stage of observation are listed. There are 12 observations within a 12-hour period from 9:00 in the morning to 8:00 at night. There is one observation, which takes only a few seconds to complete, every hour on the hour. The behaviors to be noted and their numerical codes also are listed. Each of the situations where the observations occur is indicated by two letters. Finally, the time and the number of the particular are interval shown. At 12:00, when Observation 4 occurred, Robert was seen paying attention to his work while he was sitting in the classroom. This form may be revised to reveal what task Robert was performing and in which part of the classroom; a tremendous amount of detailed information may be obtained with the time sampling technique.

The equipment necessary to observe behavior by these three techniques can be found in most variety and sporting-goods stores. Usually, all that is required are paper, pencils, a clipboard, a wrist counter, and a regular watch or a stopwatch.

Figure 2
Illustration of a time sampling recording form depicting the frequency of several behaviors in various situations for one nine-year-old boy.

Name and Age of Patient:	Robert P., 9 years old
Date of Observation:	September 4
Stage of Observation:	Baseline
Number of Observations:	12
Total Time of Observations:	12 hours

Behaviors Observed and Code

Talking to others	1
Hitting	2
Resting by lying down	3
Paying attention to task	4
Sitting	5

Situations Where Behaviors Were Observed and Code

Cafeteria	Ca
Dormitory	Do
Playroom	Pl
Classroom	Cl

Observation	Number and Time	Behaviors and Situation	
1.	9:00 a.m.	3	Do
2.	10:00 a.m.	2	Ca
3.	11:00 a.m.	2	Pl
4.	12:00 a.m.	4 - 5	Cl
5.	1:00 p.m.	1 - 2	Cl
6.	2:00 p.m.	1	Cl
7.	3:00 p.m.	1	Pl
8.	4:00 p.m.	3	Do
9.	5:00 p.m.	1	Ca
10.	6:00 p.m.	1	Pl
11.	7:00 p.m.	1	Pl
12.	8:00 p.m.	1	Do

(All data are fictitious.)

Summarizing Recorded Observations by Graphing

After observations have been gathered during baseline or during intervention stages of a behavior modification program, it is wise to summarize the notes so that correct conclusions can be made regarding such considerations as the stability of baseline or whether the procedures being used in treatment are working properly.

The most convenient recapitulation of behavior is presented by a line graph. Although there are two types which behavior modifiers use (e.g., conventional and cumulative), we will discuss only conventional diagrams.

A line graph shows the relationships between two variables; for behavior modification, they generally are time and the frequency of behavior. Time is represented along the horizontal axis (the abscissa) and frequency is represented along the vertical axis (the ordinate). Therefore, each point on the graph represents the frequency of a particular activity at a particular time (e.g., 30 hits on Day 1).

Let us consider the hypothetical case of Arnold, a 21-year-old retarded male, who lives in an institution for the mentally deficient. Generally, Arnold is not a problem for the nurses, but lately he has been leaving his bed at night. Preliminary observation reveals that Arnold gets up frequently; and each time he does so, he walks to the night nurse's office. She generally responds to Arnold's behavior by coaxing him to go back to bed.

To obtain an accurate count of Arnold's getting up, the nurses record its frequency for one week. They make no attempt to change anything. Let us say the following baseline record is obtained: on Monday Arnold gets up 9 times; on Tuesday, 12 times; on Wednesday, 11 times; on Thursday, 25 times; on Friday, 15 times; on Saturday, 12 times; on Sunday, 15 times.

Furthermore, suppose that on the basis of these seven days of observation, the nurses suggest that Arnold's getting up is being positively reinforced, inadvertently, by the attention he receives when he awakens. Consequently, the nurses attempt a simple Extinction procedure. Briefly, all the night nurses are asked to ignore Arnold's arising unless something is apparently wrong; that is, the nurses are asked to attempt no longer to coax Arnold back to bed and to stop paying excessive attention to his behavior. If he awakens, he is told only once to please return to bed. In particular, the Thursday-night nurse, who works only one night a week and who spends a great deal of time persuading Arnold to return to his bed, is asked to ignore his leaving it. This procedure is implemented for 18 days.

Thus a total of 25 days of observation are made concerning Arnold's getting-up behavior. The first 7 days consist of baseline, and the next 18 constitute Extinction treatment. All the observations may be summarized in table form. But to easily picture both the stability of baseline and the effectiveness of treatment, a graph should be made.

Figure 3 was constructed for these purposes. Time, that is, the number of days, is depicted along the horizontal axis; the numbers run from one to 25 (only the even numbers are written out, but each hatch mark stands for one day). The frequency of getting-up behavior is depicted along the vertical axis; the numbers along it begin with zero and end with 26 (again only the even numbers are written out). Twenty-six is slightly higher than the highest recorded frequency of this behavior (i.e., 25). Every point on the graph represents how often the activity occurred on that day (i.e., Day 5, 15 times; and Day 21, 0 times). To show change from day to day, the points are connected by straight lines.

Notice that each axis is labeled—Frequency, Days—and the figure has a caption and a number. In addition, each stage of the graph is labeled—Baseline, Extinction. If more than one behavior were diagramed, different kinds of lines or connection points could be used, such as dashed or dotted lines. Which specific behavior each line represents should be labeled in the corner of the diagram so that the reader knows exactly what he is seeing. A graph should tell a complete story.

From Figure 3, it appears that the baseline is fairly stable and that during the first few days of Extinction an increase in the undesirable behavior resulted. This increase, however, was temporary and, eventually, the activity decelerated to zero.

An up-to-date account of the target behaviors may be kept by plotting data points as they become available; that is, daily graphing is recommended. A skeleton of the diagram may be constructed with both axes labeled. And then, as observational information is obtained during baseline and treatment, the points can be plotted and joined. Day-to-day changes in behaviors of the individual patient, therefore, immediately become apparent to the nurses. This result is important especially during treatment because ineffective or harmful procedures can be noticed more easily and then altered.

Figure 3
Record of Arnold's nighttime waking during Baseline and Extinction.

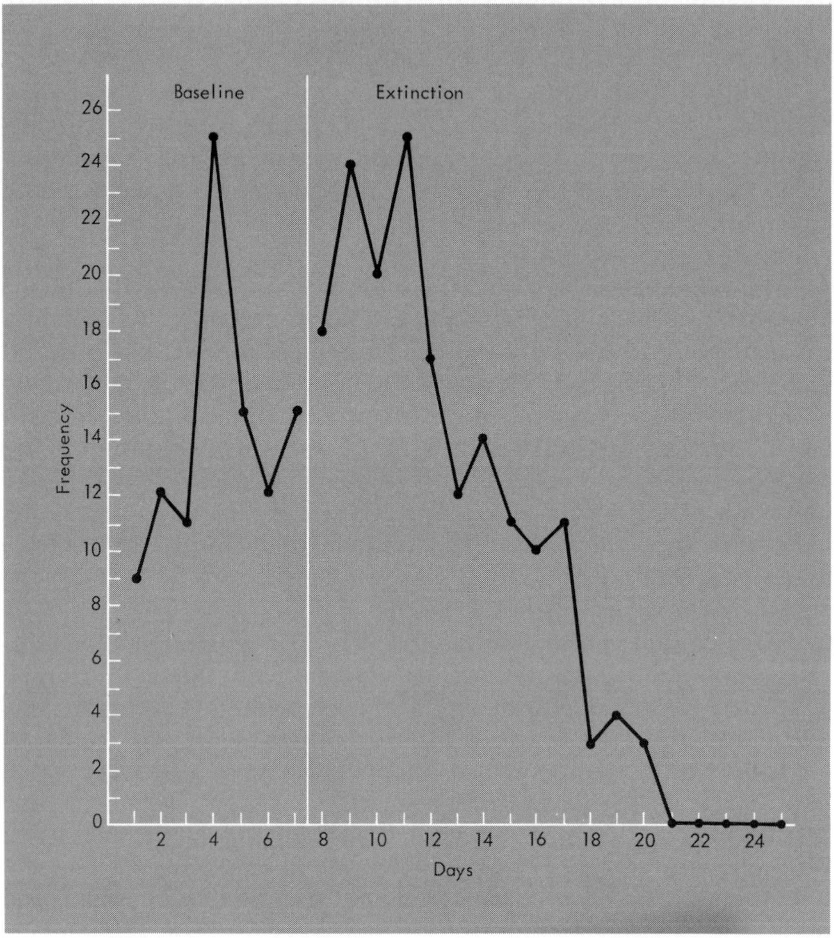

(All data are fictitious.)

Evaluating Behavior Observations

As already indicated, the first step in precisely observing and recording behavior is to define it accurately. But how confident can any nurse be that her observations will agree with some other nurse's observations of the same behavior occurring under the same conditions. To compare adequately the frequency of a patient's behavior in baseline with the frequency of his behavior both during and after intervention, the nurse must be confident that her record of observations will concur with another nurse's. Decisions about the utility of behavior modification procedures for the patient depend on accurate assessment of his behavior. Several techniques can be employed to evaluate the level or degree of agreement between two monitors.

How much concurrence exists between observers about the frequency of an individual's behavior that each has observed and has recorded at the same time is called reliability and can be expressed as a *percentage of agreement.* The higher the percentage, the greater the agreement between observers.

For example, suppose two nurses record the frequency of a behavior (e.g., the number of refusals made by a mental patient in one day). Let us say that each nurse records this patient's refusal behavior as it occurs. If Nurse A counts 22 of these activities, and Nurse B counts 23, the nurses are not in perfect concurrence. But they are close to it. Just how close can be easily determined by dividing the record of the nurse with the *lower count* (i.e., 22) *by* the record of the nurse with the *higher count* (i.e., 23). A percentage of agreement can be obtained if this result is multiplied by 100.

Thus, if just the total frequency of a behavior is recorded, the percentage of agreement between observers can be determined by the following formula:

$$\text{Percentage of agreement} = \frac{\text{record of observer with lower count}}{\text{record of observer with higher count}} \times 100$$

In this example:

$$\text{Percentage of agreement} = (22/23) \times 100 = 95.6\%$$

Since 100% is the highest possible percentage of agreement, it is safe to conclude that these two nurses concurred highly about how many times the patient's refusal behavior occurred in one day.

When interval or time sampling recording procedures are used, a different method for determining the percentage of agreement between observers is employed. The number of intervals in which nurses are in accordance that the behavior has occurred are compared.

Suppose, for example, that two nurses observed the paraplegic patient discussed above for sustained exercising. Observations by each nurse were carried out during the same five-second intervals.

Figure 4

Illustration of an interval-recording form depicting the frequency of sustained exercising for a 30-year-old patient as set down by two nurses.

Name and Age of Patient:	John O., 30 years old
Date of Observation:	September 2
Stage of Observation:	Baseline
Period and Time of Observation:	2 at 2:00 p.m.
Behavior Observed:	Exercising
Number of Intervals Observed:	24
Length of Each Interval:	5 seconds
Total Time of Observation:	2 minutes

Interval Number	Interval Score (Nurse A)	Interval Score (Nurse B)	Disagreement
1	E*	E	
2	E	E	
3	E	E	
4	I**	I	
5	E	E	
6	E	E	
7	E	E	
8	I	I	
9	I	I	
10	E	E	
11	I	I	
12	E	E	
13	E	E	
14	I	E	D***
15	I	I	
16	E	E	
17	I	I	
18	I	I	
19	E	E	
20	E	E	
21	E	E	
22	E	I	D
23	I	I	
24	I	I	

*E = interval wherein exercising was sustained for at least four seconds.

**I = interval wherein exercising was interrupted for more than one second (exercising was not sustained for at least four seconds).

***D = a disagreement between observers as to the interval score (i.e., E or I).

(All data are fictitious.)

Therefore, Figure 4 is exactly the same as Figure 1, except that the observations of a second nurse are recorded.

In Figure 4, which contains 24 intervals of five seconds each totaling two minutes of observation time, either an *E* (exercise) or an *I* (interruption) is recorded. It is evident that Nurse A and Nurse B agree almost perfectly; that is, in only two intervals (14 and 22) do they disagree about what they observed.

The percentage of agreement can be determined by the following formula:

$$\text{Percentage of agreement} = \frac{\text{number of intervals of agreement}}{\text{number of intervals of agreement} + \text{disagreement}} \times 100$$

In this case, the nurses disagreed only twice in 24 intervals. They agreed 22 times. Thus:

$$\text{Percentage of agreement} = \frac{22}{22 + 2} \times 100 = 91.6\%$$

Eighty percent shows an adequate degree of agreement. Although no absolute standards are, as yet, available (Hall, 1970), nurses should strive to attain levels of no less than 80%. Practice at observing behavior can help nurses to make more reliable observations.

TERMS AND QUESTIONS

Terms

Recording the frequency of behaviors as they occur

Interval recording

Time sampling recording

Conventional line graph

Reliability

Percentage of agreement

Questions

1. When do you use interval recording instead of simply recording the frequency of the behavior as it occurs?

2. What is the main difference between time sampling and interval recording techniques?
3. What generally is depicted along the abscissa of a behavior modification graph and along the ordinate?
4. What does each point represent on such a graph?
5. Nurse A observes that Mark P., a mental patient, leaves and returns to the daily ward meetings the following number of times:

		Nurse A	Nurse B observes the same behavior the following number of times:
1.	Monday	5	5
2.	Tuesday	6	6
3.	Wednesday	4	4
4.	Thursday	7	6
5.	Friday	8	8
6.	Saturday	10	9
7.	Monday	4	4
8.	Tuesday	4	3
9.	Wednesday	8	8
10.	Thursday	5	4

(a) Plot Nurse A's record on a graph.

(b) Over the 10 days, Nurse A counts 61 of the leaving-returning behaviors; that is, the patient left and returned to the ward meetings 61 times in 10 days, at least according to Nurse A. What does Nurse B observe?

(c) What is the percentage of agreement between Nurse A and Nurse B as to the *total* number of behaviors observed to occur?

(Let us say that the only information you have is the total frequency count of each nurse.)

5.4 *BEING SKILLFUL IN DESIGNING A BEHAVIOR MODIFICATION PROGRAM AND BEING CRITICAL IN EVALUATING THE BEHAVIOR MODIFICATION PROCEDURES*

There are four questions that the skillful and critical nurse must answer in order to create and to evaluate a behavior modification program. They are as follows: *Where do I begin? Where do I want to finish? How do I proceed from start to finish? How do I know that the procedures I have used are responsible for the behavior changes I have found?* By knowing how to observe and how to record behavior, how to apply behavior modification procedures, and how to evaluate observations and procedures, a nurse can answer these four questions.

Establishing the Starting and Finishing Points of a Behavior Modification Program (Information Pertinent to Questions 1 and 2)

A behavior modification program begins with the patient's problem and ends with a change in it. Both the beginning point and the end point must be phrased in *behavioral* terms. Clearly phrased objective statements are vital.

To say that Johnny is an isolated child and that you want to help him to become united with his peers are general statements that must be reformulated into behavioral language. If Johnny is an isolated child, he acts in certain ways that are summarized by the term *isolated*. What isolated means in Johnny's case must be defined accurately.

In order to establish which behaviors we want to change or to bring about and in what direction we want to change them, we need adequate definitions of the patient's behaviors and knowledge of their frequency and of the events that affect them.

Implementing any behavior modification procedure, therefore, is predicated on detailed information. Although this base has been mentioned previously, particularly in the last three sections of this chapter, it will be reviewed below in a condensed form:

Define the Problem. After the initial complaint that something is wrong with a particular individual's behavior (e.g., he is aggressive, or he lacks self-esteem), a preliminary observation period can be implemented. As discussed, the purpose of preliminary observation is to define the specific behaviors about which the complaint is a summarizing statement. Thus, a patient may be described as depressed all the time. After a preliminary observation period, we can identify and can define some of the specific activities that make up the general term *depressed*.

Measure the Behavior(s) to Be Altered. How strong or how weak are the behaviors we feel that we must modify (i.e., must accelerate or must decelerate)? Frequency is the most convenient measurement of behavior, but duration (i.e., how long an activity lasts) also may be used. (Which of these two measurements is employed depends, of course, on the information the observer desires.) In most cases, frequency is the measurement used, and the remainder of this discussion will involve it.

Precise measurement of behavior is aided by one or more of the recording techniques mentioned in the previous section. The record of the frequency of the behavior(s) before treatment begins is called baseline. The baseline of each behavior to be modified must be recorded. By registering an adequate baseline of the target behavior, the nurse can monitor more carefully the effects of the behavior modification procedure on it during treatment. Thus, benign or harmful methods can be remedied quickly. In other words, by comparing the frequency of the behavior before any attempts are made to modify it with the frequency of the behavior during treatment, the nurse can ascertain whether the program appears to be working.

Record Events That May Affect the Behavior. The events preceding and following a behavior can affect it. The contingency involved in the Positive Reinforcement procedure is based on making certain events the result of certain behaviors. It is difficult to know always which events are setting the occasion for a behavior and which ones may function as positive reinforcers or punishers for it, but an attempt to find out should be made. Events such as the behavior of another person, may set the occasion for the problem being measured. If the nurse observes that a particular setting or event consistently precedes the occurrence of the behavior being measured, it is likely that the event is setting the occasion for the behavior. For example, the caustic comments of one nurse may be setting the occasion for the "aggressive" behavior of a particular patient. If it is observed that this patient's "aggressive" behavior is relatively confined to this one situation (this one nurse's behavior), attempts to reduce his offensiveness should include efforts to remedy the nurse's behavior. Relatedly, there may be situations preventing the occurrence of desirable behavior. Thus, if an expectant mother, recently discharged from a hospital, is not following a prescribed diet, it may be her financial condition more than anything else that prevents her from purchasing the required foods. This antecedent factor must be considered in any attempt to modify the dietary activities of this woman.

Events following the target behavior being measured, notably the behavior of other people, may be functioning as positive reinforcers which maintain the patient's very frequent undesirable activity. Or these events may be inhibiting his infrequent desirable behavior. Sometimes by merely *rearranging* consequences (see Chapter 3, Section 3.6), the target behavior can be modified. Thus, events which rather consistently seem to follow the behavior measured should be noted.

COMPLETE THE PICTURE. A complete picture of a patient's activities includes not only his desirable and undesirable behaviors but also the behaviors that are related to them. Thus, if the goal of a behavior modification program were to accelerate Behavior C, and performing Behavior C involved Behaviors A and B, then an assessment of the patient's ability to perform these two necessary activities should be made. For example, the prerequisites of learning to cross a street on a green light and stopping on a red light include, among other behaviors, the ability to discriminate red from green. To successfully teach a retarded child to cross a busy street, depends, in part, on his ability to discriminate these two colors. If for some reason the child cannot form this discrimination, other methods must be used to teach him to cross the street. Knowledge that the child cannot discriminate red from green, therefore, would be useful information in this example.

Similarly, before some desirable target behaviors can be accelerated, competing undesirable behaviors may have to be decelerated. Thus, to increase a child's appropriate play activities, his physical assaults toward others should be decelerated first (e.g., Bijou, 1965). The frequencies of the undesirable and of the appropriate play activities must be recorded and must be altered. In short, a complete picture of the patient's problems also includes observing and recording behaviors related to the target behavior(s) being measured.

FIND POTENTIAL REINFORCERS FOR ACCELERATING BEHAVIOR. The importance of the Positive Reinforcement procedure has been discussed in both Chapters 3 and 4; even if the problem involves undesirable behavior, which must be reduced, Positive Reinforcement can be employed valuably. Consequently, the nurse should ascertain what objects or activities the patient enjoys in order that these may be used in a behavior modification program.

Information about potential reinforcers can be obtained from interviews with the patient and his family. Or the patient can be observed and the activities he frequently engages in (e.g., going to movies or being a leader of a group) can be recorded. Recall that frequently occurring activities can function as positive reinforcers if made contingent on specified desirable behavior(s). The use of tokens with these activity reinforcers also is useful (see Chapter 3, Section 3.2).

CLEARLY STATE THE GOALS OF THE BEHAVIOR MODIFICATION PROGRAM. When a nurse knows precisely what the problem is, that is, when she has an adequate baseline of particular activities and information on contributing conditions, the goals of behavior modification can be formulated exactly. These objectives represent the changes desired in particular behaviors occurring under specified conditions. Thus, if a mental patient frequently swears, especially when he encounters nurses, a goal of behavior modification would be to decelerate this behavior and to accelerate more socially appropriate verbalizations. The statements to be decelerated and the kinds of statements to be accelerated, as well as when each can or should occur, must be indicated clearly.

An accurate and precise description of the patient's behaviors helps to suggest the changes that should be made. Thus, someone described as lazy may be slow to get out of bed in the morning, may refuse to engage in any work, and may refuse occupational therapy. By knowing the behavioral referents of the term *lazy*, the nurse can formulate goals—changes in the patient's behaviors—that will improve his functioning. One objective, therefore, may be to accelerate the patient's going to occupational therapy wherein many positive reinforcers are present.

In other words, vague descriptions of goals do not suggest the changes that must be made to help a patient to behave more capably. As Schaefer and Martin (1969) point out:

> Often nursing personnel have to construct a treatment plan for inner states of the patient. For example, suppose a psychiatrist recommends that a patient's self-esteem should be "enhanced." This request should prompt the question, "What must a patient do so that you can conclude he has gained in self-esteem?" The answer to this question can only be stated in behavioral terms. Self-esteem might involve behaviors like verbal statements of achievement or statements regarding positive feelings about oneself, or it might show itself in the patient no longer mingling with groups of lower status and seeking the company of higher-status groups. Once the behavioral meaning of concepts like self-esteem are clarified, nurs-

ing personnel can formulate plans because they now have direct access to a set of behaviors.[2]

By carefully delineating the goals to be attained (Reese, 1966), the nurse is in an improved position to implement effective behavior modification procedures.

Attaining the Goals of a Behavior Modification Program (Information Pertinent to Question 3)

After observing and recording a patient's behavior and after clearly stating which activities are to be changed as well as the direction of change (i.e., acceleration, deceleration), the nurse can formulate a plan of treatment. Many of the behavior modification procedures useful in changing behavior have already been discussed. The information necessary in designing a behavior modification program utilizing these procedures is listed below:

(1) *Clearly specify the target behaviors (i.e., both* Ta *and* Td*) to be changed.* This practice was discussed above.

(2) *Designate the behavior modification procedures and all their elements to be applied to each target behavior.* For example, if the Positive Reinforcement method is to be applied to a specific behavior with a low frequency of occurrence, the types of reinforcers to be used must be defined (e.g., food, tokens, activities, and praise) and what they consist of (e.g., ice cream or a movie). In addition, the particular combinations of the reinforcers to be employed (e.g., tokens and praise) as well as the transition from one, such as food, to the other, such as praise, should be included in the description of the behavior modification procedure. Once a program is designed, however, it should be changed if it is not working well. Careful planning in advance is necessary; but blind allegiance to the project proving to be detrimental to the patient's welfare is, of course, ridiculous.

A major reason for carefully designating the behavior modification procedure to be used and for defining all its elements is to eliminate ambiguity in carrying out the program. When the exact relationship between a particular behavior and a particular consequence

---

[2]Halmuth H. Schaefer and Patrick L. Martin, *Behavioral Therapy* (New York: McGraw-Hill Book Company, 1969), p. 83.

is specified, then all of the nurses involved in treating the patient will know clearly what activity is to be followed by which consequence. Thus, if cleanliness (a behavior) is to be reinforced with tokens, the components of cleanliness (e.g., clean nails, clean shirt) that result in reinforcement (e.g., one token for each element) should be specified. In addition, the definition of clean (e.g., all the fingernails must be dirt free, and no spots or dirt may be present on the shirt) should be indicated.

Finally, as part of a complete description of behavior modification procedures, the adjunctive techniques to be used (e.g., Shaping, Instructing) should be outlined.

(3) *Indicate the frequency with which the behavior modification procedure is to be applied to the target behavior.* For example, if a Positive Reinforcement procedure is to be used, the schedule of reinforcement must be indicated (e.g., continuous reinforcement). When the behavior reaches a high frequency, an intermittent schedule should be applied in order to increase the behavior's durability. In this regard, the type of intermittent schedule of reinforcement to be used (e.g., variable ratio or variable interval) should be specified. If deceleration procedures are employed, such as Aversive Stimulation or Withdrawal of Positive Reinforcement, each occurrence of the undesirable behavior throughout the program should be followed by the presentation of the aversive stimulus or the withdrawal of the positive reinforcer.

(4) *Describe the settings where behavior modification procedures will be implemented.* The settings in which baseline records of the target behavior are obtained should be specified. At least initially, these are the circumstances where behavior modification procedures should be implemented. Furthermore, the settings where behavior modification takes place, should be the ones where the undesirable target behavior is likely to occur and where the desirable target behavior should occur. Thus, it is nonsensical to try to measure and to try to increase the frequency of social interactions when the patient is alone; also, it is foolish to attempt to increase them when he is in settings where these behaviors are undesirable (e.g., the library). Relatedly, a behavior should be accelerated in an environment conducive to its growth (Reese, 1966). For example, you should not attempt to accelerate articulate speech in a noisy room.

(5) *Specify the situations under which the target behavior must occur before it will be followed by a positive reinforcer, by an aversive stimulus, or by any other consequence.* Thus, the events that should *precede* the behavior in order for it to be reinforced have to be stated in advance. Similarly, the events that the behavior

should not be reinforced under have to be stated. Thus, if a nurse wants to accelerate a patient's social activities, she may reinforce the patient for talking, but only when he is conversing with others. If the patient is visibly with other patients, this situation is one in which talking behavior should be followed by the positive reinforcer. When the patient is not noticeably with other patients, talking behavior, if it occurs, should not be followed by the reinforcer. And in circumstances, such as a movie, even though the patient is with other patients, talking behavior also should not be reinforced.

A nurse may want to reinforce a retarded child for "paying attention." Consequently, only when the child is looking at the materials on his desk or at the nurse who is talking, should his fixated gaze be followed by a reinforcer. In other words, the fixated gazing behavior should be reinforced, only if it occurs under certain conditions. If the child were staring at an empty desk or into space, a reinforcer would not be administered. The conditions under which a behavior must occur to be reinforced have to be indicated.

(6) *Describe the materials to be used.* The recording forms for monitoring the patient's behavior and the necessary equipment (e.g., clocks and counters) should be described.

(7) *Select the agents of behavior change.* The individuals to be responsible for the various activities in a behavior modification program, such as monitoring the behavior, reinforcing it, and keeping up-to-date records should be named to avoid confusion. The nurses may wish to include other helping agents (see Chapter 3, Section 3.6). If so, their activities should be indicated clearly.

The statements made in reference to setting goals and to for mulating procedures in behavior modification reflect the specificity necessary in designing a behavior modification program for an individual and the skill required to implement it. No room for ambiguity, imprecision, or inaccuracy exists.

Critically Evaluating the Behavior Modification Procedures (Answering Question 4)

The need for evaluating observations, whenever they are made, in terms of determining a percentage of agreement has been discussed in Section 5.3. Furthermore, the importance of continued observation in the intervention phase of a behavior modification program has been emphasized; that is, the changes in behavior during treatment should be compared continually to the frequency of behavior previously tabulated in the baseline record in order to evaluate the ongoing effects of treatment.

In addition, techniques exist in behavior modification for evaluating whether *the specific procedures,* which have been applied, have in fact, caused the individual's behavior to change. As discussed in Chapter 2, however, controversy about the importance of this type of evaluation in a clinical setting can be found. But statements concerning the patient, such as "I believe he's better because of Treatment Y," can be changed to statements, such as "The patient is behaving more capably *because of* Treatment Y," provided that evaluative steps are taken. To advance patient care in general by reducing the likelihood of superstitiously applying remedies that have little effect (we are reinforced for using these procedures because, unfortunately, they are associated intermittently with patient improvement), the evaluation of procedures is essential. Some evaluative techniques used in behavior modification are listed below:

(1) *The reversal method.* This method has received the most objection from mental-health workers because it involves a reinstatement, even though temporary, of the behavior problem. This method of verification has been widely used, especially in early behavior modification applications and, therefore, will be reviewed. There are four steps in the reversal method. First, baseline information on the frequency of the behavior to be accelerated or to be decelerated is obtained. Second, after an adequate baseline record has been determined, the particular behavior modification procedure (e.g., Positive Reinforcement) is applied. Observations on the target behavior still are recorded. Third, the treatment procedure is removed. And a change in the target behavior from its treatment level to its pretreatment level (baseline) should occur. Thus, if the Positive Reinforcement procedure is applied to an activity for a certain amount of time, the activity will accelerate in frequency. When the positive reinforcers are removed, the behavior should return to its pretreatment level—its level before Positive Reinforcement was applied. If Positive Reinforcement was entirely responsible for the acceleration of the behavior, removing it should result in the deceleration of the behavior. Fourth, the treatment procedure is applied once again and the behavior, once again, changes in the desired direction. (The behavior should be measured throughout the program.)

There are problems in using this evaluative method. As stated, to require that the difficulty be reinstated is objectionable. In addition, the reversal method is not always suitable because some conditions, once changed by the treatment procedure, are difficult to reinstate even if the treatment procedure is removed. (Indeed, this result is one goal of meaningful behavior modification.)

(2) *The multiple-baseline method.* In contrast to the reversal approach, the multiple-baseline method (Baer, Wolf and Risley, 1968) does not require that the problem behavior be reinstated in order to evaluate the causal effectiveness of the treatment procedure. The multiple-baseline method evaluates the effectiveness of a behavior modification procedure by applying it to other activities of the patient. There are four essential steps involved in this approach. First, baseline records of more than one behavior of the patient are obtained, concurrently. For example, information on the frequency of talking, and smiling may be gathered at the same time. Second, after all the baseline data are recorded, the treatment procedure is applied to *one of these behaviors* (e.g., smiling is positively reinforced). Third, a comparison should be made, after the first target behavior is modified, between this activity and the other, as yet, unmodified one. Thus, the changed frequency of smiling may be compared to the unchanged frequency of talking. Because smiling has been altered, a difference between how often smiling occurs after treatment in comparison to before treatment (baseline) should be apparent. *But the frequency of talking should be unaltered.* Fourth, the behavior modification procedure is then applied to the second behavior (e.g., talking). After a change in this behavior has been found, a third and, as yet, unchanged one may also be altered. Thus, confidence in the effectiveness of the behavior modification procedure is obtained *progressively* by noting the change that occurs in each activity as the procedure is applied to it.

(3) *The differential reinforcement method.* This approach also does not require the reinstatement of the problem behavior. With the differential reinforcement method of evaluation, confidence that the behavior modification procedure has been responsible for the changed behavior is acquired by applying the procedure to another aspect or component of the target behavior; that is, the change in the target behavior is *refined* by further uses of the treatment procedure. This method is illustrated best by an example: Acker and his associates (1970) used Positive Reinforcement to accelerate speech in a 3½-year-old boy. The child's linguistic sounds increased. To evaluate this procedure and to improve the boy's speaking, Positive Reinforcement was applied to the child's *clear* statements in contrast to simple linguistic sounds that were difficult to recognize. From this second application of Positive Reinforcement, the authors found that clear word sounds increased and unclear ones decreased.

Thus, the treatment procedure was evaluated by reapplying it to a specific aspect of the original target behavior (i.e., first it was applied to speech sounds and then to intelligible words). The changes recorded in these behaviors occurred each time the procedure was implemented.

Regardless of which evaluative method is used, a follow-up period of observation of the modified behavior should be made. The *immediate* effectiveness of the procedures used should be evaluated and their *long-term* effects should be ascertained. Without information about the durability of change, the meaningfulness of a behavior change program is in doubt. Thus, after treatment has ended (e.g., three months, six months, or longer), an attempt to observe and to record the behaviors of the patient that were previously the targets of treatment should be made. In addition, new activities, both desirable and undesirable, that have arisen should be noted. The follow-up period is the most neglected. Behavior modifiers know that they can change behavior rapidly, but verified demonstrations of long-term changes are still relatively rare.

TERMS AND QUESTIONS

Terms

Reversal method
Multiple-baseline method
Differential reinforcement method

Questions

1. What information do you need to begin and to end behavior modification programs?
2. Suppose you want to design a behavior modification program to accelerate a patient's self-esteem. What information do you need in order to *implement* the Positive Reinforcement procedure to achieve this goal?
3. If you were to employ the multiple-baseline method to evaluate whether the Positive Reinforcement procedure was responsible for increasing a patient's self-esteem, what would you do?
4. Do you feel it is important to evaluate whether treatment procedures are responsible for treatment gains? If so, why? If not, why not?
5. Why are follow-up observations important?

5.5 A SYNTHESIS

This chapter has explained the techniques necessary for designing and for evaluating a behavior modification program. In particular, defining, observing and recording behavior—assessing behavior—have been discussed.

To assess behavior and the events affecting it, to implement behavior modification procedures, and to appraise effectiveness, requires that the nurse-practitioner be accurate, precise, and critical. These qualities are essential for skillfully creating and evaluating behavior modification programs.

The relationship between assessment practices and intervention ones—that is, applying behavior modification procedures to change behavior—has been shown in this chapter. Briefly, in order to implement skillfully behavior modification procedures for changing any behavior, the nurse must have already defined, observed, and recorded the behavior. In addition, to effectively monitor changes in activity during treatment, the nurse must have gathered an adequate baseline record. If behavior modification procedures are used haphazardly, without being preceded by adequate observation of the target behaviors, unwanted and perhaps harmful changes in behavior are more likely to occur unrecognized. To avoid this result, detailed information about the target behaviors and about the events affecting them should be gathered. Observation and recording must continue throughout treatment.

This chapter also has attempted to demonstrate the importance of evaluation. Without it, the nurse can never be confident that her procedures are working advantageously or that her observations agree with another nurse's. Furthermore, without evaluation, the nurse can never feel sure that the methods she has used have been the cause of the patient's improvement. The continued employment of any behavior modification procedure should be predicated on its past success. Follow-up evaluation has been mentioned as one approach to measuring whether immediate improvement in a patient's behavior is enduring; durable change is tied to meaningful behavior modification.

Generally speaking, assessment and evaluation practices seek to answer these two important questions: What do you mean when you say that the patient has a problem? How do you know that you have helped him? By explicitly showing what you mean, the practices of defining, observing and recording answer the first question (What do you mean. . . ?). By critically demonstrating the effectiveness of procedures, evaluation answers the second question (How do you know. . . ?). Not attempting to answer these questions or being prevented from answering them because of vague and imprecise statements about a patient's problem and about the ways to modify it are antithetical to productive care.

Chapters 3, 4, and 5 have presented the ways to implement behavior modification procedures, to assess behavior, and to evaluate. In short, these chapters have detailed the behavior modification process: Assessment, Intervention and Evaluation. In Chapter 6, several more applications—selected mainly because of the behavior problems they have dealt with, and not specifically because of the procedures they have used or because of the way they have employed behavior modification principles—will be demonstrated.

SUPPLEMENTARY READINGS

BIJOU, S. W., R. F. PETERSON, AND M. H. AULT "A Method to Integrate Descriptive and Experimental Field Studies at the Level of Data and Empirical Concepts," *Journal of Applied Behavior Analysis*, 1, 1968, 175–191.

DEIBERT, A. N., AND ALICE J. HARMON *New Tools for Changing Behavior.* Champaign, Illinois: Research Press, 1970, pp. 37–53.

HALL, R. V. *Behavior Management Series. Part I. Behavior Modification: The Measurement of Behavior.* Merriam, Kansas: H & H Enterprises, Inc. 1970.

REESE, ELLEN P. *The Analysis of Human Operant Behavior.* Dubuque, Iowa: Wm. C. Brown Company Publishers, 1966, pp. 49–57.

SCHAEFER, H. H., AND P. L. MARTIN *Behavioral Therapy.* New York: McGraw-Hill Book Company, 1969, pp. 65–100.

six Behavior Problems Frequently Encountered by Nurses

6.1 *APATHY*

Many mental patients are described as being apathetic because they seem to lack motivation for participating in activities or because they seem withdrawn. The term *apathetic* is a label representing the way in which the patient behaves; that is, the clinical judgment that a patient is apathetic is related to the decision about how he acts under specific circumstances.

To implement effective behavior modification programs for reducing apathy among mental hospital patients, we need an accurate definition of exactly what constitutes the descriptive term, apathy—what does a patient do or not do that leads other people to judge him stolid. Through many observations of mental patients, Schaefer and Martin (1966)[1] found that those patients described by psychiatrists, psychologists, and nurses as apathetic were likely to engage in only *one* behavior at a time. As discussed previously, these authors utilized a time sampling observation form for depicting the behaviors of mental patients on token-economy wards. Patients

[1]H.H. Schaefer and Patrick L. Martin, "Behavioral therapy for 'apathy' of hospitalized schizophrenics," *Psychological Reports*, 19, 1966, 1147–1158.

were observed at half-hour intervals, and their behaviors were recorded. A patient could be engaged in several activities at one time (e.g., sitting and smoking while watching T.V.) or he might be involved in only one at a time (e.g., either walking, running, standing, sitting, or lying down). Apathetic patients often were found engaging in only one behavior at a time. They did not evidence variety in their activities; instead, they were involved in single behaviors.

To modify apathy, therefore, it was necessary to accelerate multiple behaviors (variety). Special lists of target behaviors (tailored to each patient) and a general enumeration of target behaviors (for all patients) were designated; the general classes of behavior included activities involving personal hygiene, social interaction, and work efficiency. Tokens—the main reinforcers used—verbal praise, and other reinforcers (e.g., cigarettes) were made contingent on the occurrences of activities on both lists.

The accelerated behaviors were essential to the description of the patient as nonapathetic. In other words, the absence of these activities contributed to labeling the patient apathetic. Thus, during the program, a patient would be reinforced for saying, "Good morning," if the absence of this verbal behavior contributed to his considered indifference.

Twenty female patients labeled apathetic were given behavior modification. Twenty other female patients also considered apathetic were administered routine nursing care for their indifference; that is, at times these patients might be told to "take a little more interest," but engaging in a variety of behaviors (i.e., being nonapathetic) was not followed by tokens.

Before intervention began, baseline information on the number of times the patients were engaging in single classes of behavior was gathered—an assessment of apathy was made for the forty patients. A time sampling technique of observation and recording was implemented; the patients were observed at half-hour intervals each day (30 times per day) for five days.

After baseline, intervention (the Positive Reinforcement procedure) commenced and lasted three months. Observations were gathered twice during treatment in the same way as during baseline. Alterations in the program for each of the twenty patients given behavior modification could be made as needed because the staff met daily to discuss progress.

The results showed that apathy, as defined, was reduced. The twenty treated patients evidenced more multiple behaviors as opposed to single ones. The twenty nontreated patients, who at the start of intervention were similar to the treated patients in terms of their apathy ratings, did not show any marked changes as a function of routine hospital care. These results suggest that the behavior modification program was more successful than the conventional hospital method.

In conclusion, as the authors mentioned, changing behavior, such as apathy, that contributes to the patient's distance from the outside community helps to eventuate his successful return to it.

QUESTIONS

1. What was the behavioral definition of "apathy" used in this example?
2. How would you go about formulating a behavioral definition of exuberance in young children (e.g., 4-year-olds)?

6.2 *ANOREXIA NERVOSA*

A patient diagnosed as anorexic displays a severely reduced level of eating accompanied by a weight loss. Since such patients may evidence nutritional deficits, the condition of anorexia nervosa may be dangerous. Bachrach, Erwin, and Mohr (1965) reported a case study in which a patient lost approximately 73 pounds over a period of several years.

Leitenberg, Agras, and Thomson (1968)[2] showed how behavior modification principles were used effectively and meaningfully to help two hospitalized adolescent females (ages 14 and 17), both of whom demonstrated behaviors characteristic of anorexia nervosa—reduced eating and loss of weight. Only the procedures used for the 14-year-old patient will be described in detail.

Originally, this patient was hospitalized because of various somatic complaints (e.g., stomach discomfort, "vomiting") and because of marked weight loss. Exploratory abdominal surgery revealed no physical reason for her reports of intense discomfort. By the time the girl was transferred to the facility where the behavior modification program was implemented, she weighed 76 pounds.

Two classes of behavior were designated as the goals of treatment. The first involved the patient's physical complaints, and the

[2]Harold Leitenberg, W. Stewart Agras, and Lawrence Thomson, "A sequential analysis of the effect of selective positive reinforcement in modifying anorexia nervosa," *Behaviour Research and Therapy*, 6, 1968, 211–218.

second involved her reduced level of food intake and weight loss. To decelerate her physical complaints (her *Td*'s), an Extinction procedure was instituted; that is, the nurses ignored the patient's complaints of headaches, pains, and so forth. A rapid decline in her grumbling followed the application of this procedure. A 10-day baseline period of routine nursing care preceded the implementation of Extinction.

Extinction seemed to alter the verbal behavior of the patient, but her reduced level of eating still remained a serious problem. Consequently, a program (i.e., the Positive Reinforcement procedure) for accelerating desirable eating activities (*Ta*'s) was begun. Specific target behaviors were designated as reinforceable. They involved gradual increases both in food eaten and in weight gained. Weight gains were followed by activity reinforcers (privileges), and increments in food consumed were followed by social reinforcers (praise). The patient's daily weight, her calorie intake, and the number of mouthfuls of food she had eaten were monitored during the study. *When the patient ate more than she had done previously, she was praised; when she evidenced an increase in weight (progressively greater increments in weight were required), she was allowed to watch T.V., and so on.* A male student, present at suppertime, praised the patient when the number of mouthfuls of food that she had consumed (she counted them aloud) exceeded those found for preceding meals. In addition, the patient monitored both the frequency of mouthfuls she had taken at other meals as well as the gradual changes in her daily weight. She recorded this information on a graph. (As will be indicated in the Concluding Statement, a graph that visibly shows the patient that he is making progress toward a goal can be a reinforcer that maintains his continued efforts.) In addition to these procedures, the nurses attempted to praise the patient when she made desirable comments concerning her health and her eating behaviors.

It appeared that the results of making positive reinforcers contingent on progressive increments in weight and food eaten—Shaping desirable behaviors—were beneficial. The patient increased her calorie intake from approximately 1700 calories a day in the beginning to over 4000 calories a day by the end of the behavior modification program; in a related way, her weight increased from 75 pounds to 93 pounds. The Positive Reinforcement procedure was in operation for less than two months. Follow-up observations (after nine months) revealed that the desirable change was durable; at this time, the patient "weighed 98 pounds and was attending school regularly."

No specific evaluative technique (see Chapter 5) was employed to ascertain whether the Positive Reinforcement procedure alone had caused the desirable behavior changes. But because no other variables seemed to have any effect and because no other treatment procedures were found to alter the patient's condition (e.g., prior to behavior modification the patient had been given, "milieu therapy," "depth interviews," and "drug therapy"), it seems that the contingent use of positive reinforcers was responsible for the desirable behavior changes.

A reversal technique of evaluation (i.e., the positive reinforcers, which were contingent on the *Ta*'s, were discontinued temporarily) was, however, employed for the 17-year-old patient mentioned above. But this removal had no marked effect; that is, once the Positive Reinforcement method had been applied, its absence did not decelerate the patient's weight gains or her daily calorie intake. The authors suggested that initially after external positive reinforcers were administered contingent on this 17-year-old girl's weight gains, for example, she may have been brought into contact with other potent reinforcers—namely, "self-observed signs of progressive improvement." These success experiences might have become quite powerful. If this effect took place, the temporary removal of the external reinforcers (e.g., privileges) would have had little influence on the patient's behaviors. In other words, signs of improvement that the patient herself could discern might have become very powerful reinforcers and, therefore, could have maintained her weight gaining efforts; consequently, the removal of external reinforcers would have had little influence on the occurrences of the desirable behaviors. (Perhaps a multiple-baseline technique, instead of the reversal method, might have been used for evaluation.)

QUESTIONS

1. How was "anorexia nervosa" dealt with in Section 6.2?
2. How may the multiple-baseline technique of evaluation be used in this example?

6.3 *LACK OF SELF-SUFFICIENCY*

To build behaviors that help individuals to attain an increased degree of independence from the total care of others is certainly a worthwhile goal of treatment. Unfortunately many problems (e.g., running the psychiatric ward smoothly and the feeling that the patient cannot be taught) interfere with attempts to build self-sufficiency. The profoundly retarded child or adult, who may be incontinent, may be unable to feed himself, and may be immobile, often presents an extreme case of excessive dependency. Attempts to teach these individuals to become more self-sufficient through the judicious application of behavior modification principles have been reported in this book (e.g., Application 7).

Loynd and Barclay (1970)[3] reported the use of behavior modification principles to teach a profoundly retarded (microcephalic) eight-year-old girl to walk by herself. At the beginning of the program, the child would take a few steps but not without the support of furniture. To teach her to walk unassisted, the therapist had to administer reinforcers contingent on walking without supports—independent walking (*Ta*); that is, walking had to be accelerated, but holding onto furniture while walking had to be eliminated.

Because the child could stand and could advance a few steps while she was holding onto a table, this point was the one at which Shaping behavior began. Potent positive reinforcers were chosen (e.g., candy and other primary reinforcers) that would be administered contingent on progressive steps toward the target behavior. (Primary reinforcers are particularly useful when working with the retarded, especially if other reinforcers [e.g., praise] are impotent.)

Briefly, the essential procedures the therapist used involved making positive reinforcers contingent on greater increases in walking while gradually Fading-out the supports, that is, gradually lessening the influence or the control of the supports over the behavior. Thus, holding onto the table was replaced by holding onto a broomstick placed between two tables. (Holding onto the broomstick resulted in the administration of reinforcers while table holding did not.) Later on, broomstick holding was decelerated and taking the teacher's hand was strengthened. By this time, the child could walk forward sufficiently but not by herself. Consequently, the therapist's hand was replaced with a short stick, which was gradually attenuated in size. The stick was replaced by a small piece of tape and then by a string. Walking forward continued to be reinforced at the same time that these supports were being faded-out. Within approximately 84 teaching periods, the child learned to walk independently ("with the minimal aid of the string").

She developed the ability to perform other behaviors that were

---

[3]Jenni Loynd and A. Barclay, "A case study in developing ambulation in a profoundly retarded child," *Behaviour Research and Therapy*, 8, 1970, 207.

not accelerated purposely by the therapist. For example, the child seemed to become more responsive socially and to become better able to feed herself. In addition, the authors reported that her family has accepted her more than before.

Positive side effects such as these may be the result of increasing the child's self-sufficiency and, thereby, bringing her into contact with more of her world. As discussed in Chapter 3, Section 3.6, the development of many desirable behaviors becomes likely once the patient comes into touch with the sources of behavior modification that exist in his environment. The authors indicated that the child's parents were present during many of the teaching sessions, and that this factor probably contributed to her learning new desirable behaviors; that is, the parents were helped to learn about applying the Positive Reinforcement procedure.

Positive side effects of behavior modification programs have been found in similar studies. Miller, Patton, and Henton (1971) reported that after they had increased a profoundly retarded boy's ability to feed himself, to respond to verbal commands, and to stand without support, he evidenced a greater responsiveness to his environment. These authors observed, quite correctly, that the likelihood of desired side effects accruing from behavior modification programs is as fruitful an area of research as is the potential development of undesired side effects.

QUESTIONS

1. How would you find out what events function as positive reinforcers for a profoundly retarded child?
2. What behavior modification procedures were used in this section? How were they used?

6.4 *SOCIAL ISOLATION*

Hall and Broden (1967)[4] reported three studies, each of which demonstrated the applicability of behavior modification principles in helping brain-injured children to behave more capably. In addi-

[4] R. Vance Hall and Marcia Broden, "Behavior changes in brain-injured children through social reinforcement," *Journal of Experimental Child Psychology*, 5, 1967, 463–479.

tion, by their studies, the authors re-affirmed the feasibility of teaching parents and educators these principles.

Only one of the cases reported by Hall and Broden will be described, namely, that of a nine-year-old boy with a probable dysfunction of the central nervous system. The boy's daily activities were characterized by several undesirable behaviors, but of particular importance was his lack of social play with his peers. Usually, he would seek attention from his teachers, but he rarely would engage in play with the other children. (The boy was one of several pupils in an experimental school for children with behavior problems.)

To rectify the child's isolate behavior, the authors taught his teachers to implement effective behavior modification procedures, namely, Positive Reinforcement (Shaping) and Extinction. Before intervention was begun, however, an assessment of the child's behavior problems had been carried out: First, during five days, preliminary observations of the child's behaviors as well as of their typical social consequences were collected. Second, an adequate definition of social play was formulated. According to the authors, "Social play included parallel and cooperative play during which the [children] engaged in similar activities involving the same or similar material in proximity to each other (within 6 feet)."[5]

Third, during eight sessions, baseline information on the amount of social interaction and the events influencing this behavior was gathered during each daily play period. An interval-recording technique was used; blocks were 10 seconds long, and total observation time for any one period was 51 minutes on the average. (The degree of agreement between observers concerning what they had noted was calculated by the method outlined in Chapter 5 for interval recording; an adequate level of agreement was found throughout the program.) During baseline, the observers avoided all interaction with the child in order to assess his behaviors accurately. Baseline observations revealed that the child engaged in very little social play with his peers during each recreational period. He did, however, attempt to interact with his teachers. From the baseline information, the authors were able to suggest that the child's lack of play with his peers was being reinforced unintentionally by the attention he was receiving from his teachers.

Consequently, 19 sessions of intervention procedures were designed to redirect the teachers' use of social consequences; that is,

---

[5]Ibid., p. 473.

instead of conversing with the child when he was *not* playing with his peers, the teachers made social reinforcers contingent on appropriate play—the occurrence of this target behavior resulted in attention from the teachers.

Although the teachers initially had some difficulties in carrying out the behavior modification procedures, they eventually were able to effect an increase in the social behavior designated. (A Shaping procedure had to be utilized whereby the child's "looking," "approaching," and "playing" behaviors were followed by reinforcers.) Three sessions of a reversal method of evaluation were used after the target behavior was noticeably increased; when positive reinforcers no longer followed the child's playing with his peers, this target behavior rapidly decelerated. Positive Reinforcement caused the desirable behavior changes. This effective procedure was reintroduced for seven additional sessions, which resulted in the return of the target behavior to a high level.

At the end of the behavior modification program, some additional desirable behavior changes were observed (e.g., the child demonstrated increased cooperation in other enterprises).

After 90 days, a follow-up period of observation was conducted. What was noted during it showed that the desirable change in the target behavior—increased play with peers—was durable and was occurring in a different setting from before (i.e., the child was transferred to a special public school). As mentioned by the authors and as discussed previously, the contact that this child eventually was able to make with his peers, once he learned to interact with them more frequently, probably helped in extending the durability and breadth of desirable behavior change.

In sum, these authors were able to teach others to administer social reinforcers effectively in order to alter the social isolation of a brain-injured child. Other reports are available which show that social reinforcers can be used to modify extreme isolation. Milby (1970), for example, discussed how the social behaviors of two isolated male patients were increased through the contingent administration of approval by the treatment staff of a psychiatric ward.

QUESTIONS

1. What were the assessment, intervention, and evaluation methods used in this section?

2. Do you believe that the example of "Social Isolation" is a well-designed behavior modification program? If so, why? If not, why not?

6.5 *OBJECTIONABLE PATTERNS OF EATING*

Undesirable patterns of eating can be one of several time-consuming management problems that confront nursing personnel who take care of retarded adults, adolescents, and children; but these eating behaviors can be decelerated in a minimum amount of time. As mentioned previously, many behavior problems of the retarded (e.g., lack of smiling) contribute to their being separated from the rest of society and to their being seen as less than human. Problems such as these must be focused on when teaching programs are formulated for these individuals.

With what seems to be a minimum amount of effort, Barton et al. (1970)[6] taught the staff of a cottage for retarded men (ages 9–23) to implement Withdrawal of Positive Reinforcement procedures (Time-Out). The goal was to decelerate the undesirable eating behaviors of 16 residents. After a preliminary observation period, several behaviors could be defined which composed the entire meal-time activity. Four of them, namely, "stealing," "using fingers inappropriately," "messy use of utensils," and "pigging," were designated as target behaviors (*Td*).

Observations during baseline and intervention were gathered for each of the 16 residents of the cottage at both lunch and dinner. Each resident was observed for either 10 seconds or until he engaged in one of the target behaviors. After all the individuals who were eating had been monitored once in this fashion, the observational technique was repeated; according to the authors, each person was observed from one-half dozen to a dozen times at each meal. The degree of agreement between observers concerning what they had seen was high throughout the study. (Although observations were gathered during lunch and during dinner, the behavior modification procedures were implemented for all three meals.)

---

[6]Elizabeth S. Barton, Doug Guess, Eugene Garcia, and Donald M. Baer, "Improvement of retardates' mealtime behaviors by time-out procedures using multiple baseline techniques," *Journal of Applied Behavior Analysis*, 3, 1970, 77–84.

Two different time-out procedures were employed. One of them required that the individual be removed from the meal for its duration (i.e., he was asked to go or was placed in a time-out room devoid of positive reinforcers). The other time-out method entailed the removal of the individual's food tray for 15 seconds only. Both approaches were used on a behavior-contingent basis; that is, when the patient engaged in "stealing," for example, he was put in the time-out room; or when he engaged in "pigging," his food tray was immediately removed for 15 seconds.

The 15-second time-out was used with more frequently occurring target behaviors (i.e., "pigging," "messy use of utensils") because it was felt that they required additional treatment. (This time-out procedure also was employed with five of the residents who used their "fingers inappropriately" because depriving them of their total meal was considered injurious.)

After six months of the behavior modification program, each of the target behaviors was noticeably less frequent: each of them had decelerated to almost zero. But no individual had lost a significant amount of weight. Furthermore, other desirable activity, namely, using eating utensils appropriately increased in frequency (as "messy use of utensils" decreased), although no specific attempt to accelerate that class of behavior was made.

Each of the four target behaviors, beginning with "stealing" and ending with "pigging," was markedly decelerated *only* when the time-out procedure was applied to it. First, the time-out procedure was used to decelerate stealing. When this behavior appeared to be decreasing, time-out was applied to the next, as yet, unchanged behavior ("using fingers inappropriately"). As soon as this second activity changed, the third one was dealt with ("messy use of utensils"). Note that time-out remained in use for each target behavior once the procedure was applied; for example, time-out continued to be used for "stealing" even after the method had begun to be applied to "using fingers inappropriately."

By sequentially applying time-out to each target behavior, the authors and the cottage staff were able to evaluate whether time-out caused the undesirable behaviors to decelerate. Because each target behavior changed *only* after time-out had been applied to it, not before, it was possible to conclude that time-out was responsible for the alterations. This type of evaluation, as discussed, is the multiple baseline method.

In sum, with the aid of essentially simple behavior modification procedures, the eating activities of 16 retarded individuals were improved.

QUESTIONS

1. If the reversal method of evaluation would have been used in this example, what problems could have arisen?
2. How may the Positive Reinforcement procedure be used in this example?

6.6 *CHRONIC PAIN*

Fordyce et al. (1968),[7] as mentioned in Chapter 1, showed how a rehabilitation team composed of nurses, physiatrists, social workers, rehabilitation counselors, and psychologists effectively reduced the chronic pain activities of three hospitalized patients by systematically applying behavior modification principles. The cooperation of the patient and his family was enlisted in an effort to extend the in-hospital treatment to the home environment. In general, family members were taught during weekly sessions to administer praise sincerely contingent on the patient's desirable behaviors, to be neutral when the patient acted undesirably, and to record precisely instances of selected target behaviors—family members were taught some basic behavior modification practices; during the program, the patient, also, was instructed to record his own behavior.

The authors mentioned that there exist many possible causes of pain. Frequently, pain-ridden individuals are helped through efforts to remove the physical causes of their discomfort. At times, however, these efforts prove unsuccessful; that is, some individuals who report to have been suffering from pain for many years (e.g., the individuals treated in the present study) have not been helped effectively by the attempts to search for underlying causes. For these people, the authors have provided an alternative approach to treatment, namely, behavior modification; this strategy focuses on the pain behaviors directly—pain behaviors that, for individuals suffering from chronic pain, are likely to have been learned. The authors

[7]Wilbert Fordyce, Roy S. Fowler, Justus F. Lehmann, Barbara J. Delateur, "Some implications of learning in problems of chronic pain," *Journal of Chronic Diseases*, 21, 1968, 179–190.

are careful to point out that behavior modification is neither applicable to all cases of chronic pain nor is it implemented effectively without considering the medical factors in each case. (The behavior modification programs for the three patients reported in this article were monitored by physicians and physiatrists at all times.)

To design effective behavior modification programs, the authors had to ascertain the behaviors characteristically engaged in by individuals who reported chronic pain. Target behaviors (both *Ta* and *Td*) then could be formulated. Pain behaviors entailed such activities as moaning, grimacing, and requesting the help of others. Generally, target behaviors to be reduced included the patient's *use of narcotics to relieve pain* and his *lack of productive activities when he reported pain* (e.g., "reclining," "halting work until the pain abates"). Target behaviors to be accelerated included the patient's engaging in *behaviors (e.g., working efficiently and walking) incompatible with nonproductive ones.*

When possible, pain behaviors (e.g., the patient's complaints about pain) were not followed by attention, whereas adaptive behaviors (e.g., walking) were followed by social reinforcers. Thus, an attempt was made throughout the behavior modification program to ignore undesirable behaviors and to reinforce desirable ones.

The frequency with which the patient took pain-killing drugs was decelerated by no longer administering them contingent on his report of pain, by gradually decreasing the narcotic content of each dosage that was dispensed, and by gradually reducing the number of medication administrations per se. First, instead of giving the patient the medicines when he reported pain, the staff administered them at regular intervals, regardless of the patient's report. Because receipt of drugs could function to strengthen the patient's reporting pain (i.e., drugs provide relief, and the administration of drugs by the staff is one form of social attention), the contingency between reporting pain and receiving drugs was disrupted—drugs were given but *not* because the patient reported pain. Second, the time between drug administrations was gradually lengthened. Finally, the analgesic content of each drug administered was reduced progressively; a masking solution was employed in order to make the gradual reduction of the narcotic undetectable to the patient. (The taste, color, and amount of the narcotic could not be discerned by the patient when it was placed in the masking solution.)

Positive reinforcers (e.g., rest and attention) were made contingent on the target behaviors to be accelerated. Thus, walking progressively more each day was followed by staff attention and by the opportunity to rest. Baseline information on the patient provided the standard that the staff could use to set goals of walking for him. The patient recorded the amount of time he spent on foot and the distance he went. Also, the patient checked in at the nursing station when he began and when he finished his walks—this reporting served as a check on the accuracy of the patient's records. Both during an assigned walk and after completing one, the patient received much attention from the staff; in addition, at the end of a prescribed stroll, the patient was allowed a rest period.

A similar procedure was implemented for assigned tasks (e.g., weaving) during occupational therapy. Both the amount of effort and the time spent on the exercise were progressively increased over baseline. The therapist set goals for the patient. Rest was made contingent on the work completed, not on the report of pain.

Social reinforcers also were made to follow noticeable increases in the duration of other activities of the patient's own choosing; the patient was taught to keep accurate records of these activities.

Thus the overall objective of the behavior modification program was to accelerate behaviors incompatible with chronic pain activities at the same time as these pain activities were decelerated; the program was begun in the hospital, but then it was shifted to the patient's home.

Three patients who complained of chronic discomfort were administered tailored forms of this behavior modification program. Each of the patients made significant improvements. A 37-year-old woman, for instance, who for almost 18 years had experienced low-back pain, and who could not engage in sustained activity for longer than 20 minutes without experiencing pain, was successfully helped. Before behavior modification was attempted, however, her medical history (which revealed previous surgical operations for the "removal of a herniated disk" and for "a lumbosacral spine fusion") and her present physical condition were evaluated.

This woman's drug taking (the patient swallowed several habit forming analgesic tablets each day) was reduced markedly, and her productive-activity level was increased markedly after eight weeks of in-hospital care and 23 weeks of outpatient treatment. During the patient's stay in the hospital (at which time her husband was taught to utilize behavior modification principles), her speed of walking and the amount of distance traveled (almost two miles per day) as well as the hours of activity she spent each week were accelerated noticeably; furthermore, the active analgesic components of her medications were decreased to zero.

These positive behavior changes, accomplished by employing the behavior modification program outlined above, took place relatively quickly. And these positive alterations, as evidenced by the author's report, were durable; that is, the desirable effects of treatment, which had begun in the hospital setting, were maintained when the patient returned home—the patient has become an "independently mobile" member of her family.

QUESTIONS

1. How may behavior modification principles be incorporated in a treatment program designed to forestall the development of chronic pain behaviors (e.g., excessive reliance on drugs) in a patient suffering from a herniated disc due to a recent injury?
2. What are some of the behavior modification principles that are useful in making desirable behavior changes, which have taken place in the hospital, durable when the patient returns home? Discuss.

6.7 *DISRUPTIVE BEHAVIORS IN THE HOME*

Because any individual's behaviors (desirable and undesirable) are affected by those of others who are actively involved with him, it is often advisable to change the reactions of these other people in order to alter the individual's activities. More specifically, a person with behavior problems can be helped if the reactions to his undesirable activities from his family, teachers, or peers are changed. Thus, as indicated previously, an effective strategy for dealing with behavior problems, particularly those of people residing in the community, is to alter the reinforcement practices of the important members of the person's environment.

Hawkins et al. (1966)[8] showed that the problems (e.g., aggressiveness, disobedience, tantruming) of a four-year-old boy could be reduced when his mother's reactions were changed. Preliminary observations indicated (1) that the mother paid a good deal of attention to her child's undesirable behaviors, which probably accounted for their high frequency, and (2) that the child primarily engaged in nine different undesirable behaviors. Rather than attempting to

[8]Robert Hawkins, Robert Peterson, Edda Schweid, and Sidney Bijou, "Behavior therapy in the home: Amelioration of problem parent-child relations with the parent in a therapeutic role," *Journal of Experimental Child Psychology,* 4, 1966, 99–107.

reduce each of them individually, the authors classified them together as "Objectionable Behavior" and then attempted to reduce this class. Some of the behaviors included under the rubric Objectionable were "biting his shirt or arm," "sticking out his tongue," and "kicking or hitting himself, others or objects."

Baseline information about the frequency of undesirable behavior was gathered in 16 sessions. To record this class of activity an interval technique was used; that is, every 10 seconds the occurrence or nonoccurrence of unwanted behavior was written down. The degree of agreement regarding the observations was calculated and was found to be generally high throughout the study. (The degree of agreement between observers was calculated by the method outlined in Chapter 5 for recording the frequency of events as they occur, not by the method outlined for interval recording.) Two other classes of behavior involving the frequency of the child and mother saying something to one another also were recorded and were evaluated in the same fashion.

Each session during baseline and treatment generally lasted an hour and took place from two to three times per week. The entire behavior modification program for the child occurred *in his home* with few restrictions being placed on his movements or on the presence of various family members. In short, the child was observed and was treated in the same situation (and under the same general conditions) wherein his undesirable activities customarily took place.

Six sessions of intervention followed baseline. The objective of this stage was to teach the mother how to reduce her child's objectionable behavior. To accomplish this goal, a therapist (who was present during each treatment session) signaled the mother when to apply one of three procedures. The first time the child engaged in objectionable behavior during any given treatment session, the mother was signaled to tell her son to stop whatever he was doing. The second time the child became engrossed in obnoxious behavior and thereafter, during any given session, the mother was signaled to apply a Withdrawal of Positive Reinforcement procedure (Time-Out). The child was placed in his own room, which previously was made deficient in positive reinforcers, for at least five minutes; a time-out delay was employed (see Chapter 4, Section 4.3). The third procedure, Positive Reinforcement, required that the mother attend to, praise, and lovingly touch her son contingent on his behaving desirably; the therapist also signaled the mother exactly when to apply this method. In short, the mother was taught, not simply told, how she should react to her child in order to improve his behavior.

Intervention clearly was successful: objectionable behavior was decelerated. The difference, in terms of the maximum number of times offensive activity had occurred in one session, between baseline and treatment, was 105; that is, the maximum number of times offensive activity had occurred in one baseline session was 113, whereas the maximum number of times in one treatment session was eight. When a reversal method of evaluation, consisting of 14 sessions, was attempted (the mother was told to react to her son as she had done during baseline), only a partial return of objectionable behavior was found. According to the authors, the incomplete return of the undesirable activities was in part due to the mother's inability to react as she had done previously. The mother had difficulty in returning to her old ways. Treatment procedures were reapplied for six sessions, and a deceleration of the target behavior class resulted once again.

Follow-up observations, which were gathered after approximately one month, showed that the desirable behavior changes were durable. The child was reported to be behaving better, and the Withdrawal of Positive Reinforcement procedure was being used by the mother infrequently. In addition, the authors mentioned that the mother no longer was providing attention for her son's objectionable behavior—she had become more effective in dealing with her child.

Various studies have been reported that have re-affirmed the feasibility of conducting behavior modification programs entirely within the community (e.g., home) environment (see, LeBow, 1972). Teaching parents and others to utilize behavior modification principles effectively, can be, as has been suggested, instrumental in making behavior modification programs meaningful and in preventing the unbridled development of other behavior problems.

QUESTIONS

1. How would you have used the multiple baseline technique in this section?
2. What are some advantages of extending to, or of conducting behavior modification programs in the home?

SUPPLEMENTARY READINGS

AYLLON, T. "Intensive Treatment of Psychotic Behaviour by Stimulus Satiation and Food Reinforcement," *Behaviour Research and Therapy*, 1, 1963, 53–61.

———, AND J. MICHAEL "The Psychiatric Nurse as a Behavioral Engineer," *Journal of the Experimental Analysis of Behavior,* 2, 1959, 323–334.

AZRIN, N. H., AND R. M. FOXX "A Rapid Method of Toilet Training the Institutionalized Retarded," *Journal of Applied Behavior Analysis,* 4, 1971, 89–99.

AZRIN, N. H., H. RUBIN, F. O'BRIEN, T. AYLLON, AND D. ROLL "Behavioral Engineering: Postural Control by a Portable Operant Apparatus," *Journal of Applied Behavior Analysis,* 1, 1968, 99–108.

BACHRACH,. A. J., W. J. ERWIN, AND J. P. MOHR "The Control of Eating Behavior in an Anorexic by Operant Conditioning Techniques," in *Case Studies in Behavior Modification,* eds. L. P. Ullmann and L. Krasner. New York: Holt, Rinehart & Winston, Inc., 1965.

BRADY, J. P. "Metronome-Conditioned Speech Retraining for Stuttering," *Behavior Therapy,* 2, 1971, 129–150.

BURCHARD, J. D., AND V. O. TYLER, JR. "The Modification of Delinquent Behaviour Through Operant Conditioning," *Behaviour Research and Therapy,* 2, 1965, 245–250.

CUSHING, MARTHA "When Counseling Fails, Then What?" *Journal of Rehabilitation,* July–August, 1969, pp. 18–20.

GERICKE, O. L. "Practical Use of Operant Conditioning in a Mental Hospital," *Psychiatric Studies & Projects,* 3, 1965, 2–10.

HEWETT, F. M. "Teaching Speech to an Autistic Child Through Operant Conditioning," *American Journal of Orthopsychiatry,* 35, 1965, 927–936.

HINGTGEN, J. N., AND F. C. TROST, JR. "Shaping Cooperative Responses in Early Childhood Schizophrenics: II. Reinforcement of Mutual Physical Contact and Vocal Responses," in *Control of Human Behavior,* eds. R. Ulrich, T. Stachnik and J. Mabry. Glenview, Illinois: Scott, Foresman and Company, 1966.

LAL, H., AND O. R. LINDSLEY "Therapy of Chronic Constipation in a Young Child by Rearranging Social Contingencies," *Behaviour Research and Therapy,* 6, 1968, 484–485.

LINDSLEY, O. R. "Geriatric Behavioral Prosthetics," in *Control of Human Behavior,* eds. R. Ulrich, T. Stachnik, and J. Mabry. Glenview, Illinois: Scott, Foresman and Company, 1966.

MATHIS, H. I. "Training a 'Disturbed' Boy Using the Mother as Therapist: A Case Study," *Behavior Therapy,* 2, 1971, 233–239.

MILBY, J. B. "Modification of Extreme Social Isolation by Contingent Social Reinforcement," *Journal of Applied Behavior Analysis,* 3, 1970, 149–152.

MILLER, H. R., MARY E. PATTON, AND K. R. HENTON "Behavior Modification in a Profoundly Retarded Child: A Case Report," *Behavior Therapy,* 2, 1971, 375–384.

RICKARD, H. C., AND T. R. SAUNDERS, JR. "Control of 'Clean-Up' Behavior in a Summer Camp," *Behavior Therapy,* 2, 1971, 340–344.

Salzinger, K., R. S. Feldman, and Stephanie Portnoy "Training Parents of Brain-Injured Children in the Use of Operant Conditioning Procedures," *Behavior Therapy*, 1, 1970, 4–32.

Sulzer, E. S. "Behavior Modification in Adult Psychiatric Patients," in *Case Studies in Behavior Modification*, eds. L. P. Ullmann and L. Krasner. New York: Holt, Rinehart & Winston, Inc., 1965.

Toepfer, Caroline, Jeanette Reuter, and C. D. Maurer "The Design and Evaluation of an Obedience Training Program for Mothers of Preschool Children." Paper presented at the meeting of the Midwestern Psychological Association, Cincinnati, Ohio, 1970.

Zeilberger, Jane, Sue E. Sampen, and H. N. Sloane, Jr. "Modification of a Child's Problem Behaviors in the Home, with the Mother as Therapist," *Journal of Applied Behavior Analysis*, 1, 1968, 47–53.

seven Behavior Modification Programs for Groups of Individuals

7.1 TOKEN REINFORCEMENT PROGRAMS

General Description

Token reinforcement programs are systems of behavior modification designed to foster the adaptive behavior of relatively large *groups* of persons in institutions and other settings wherein groups of people perform similar activities. In a token program, a patient can earn tokens if he engages in certain designated behaviors and can spend his earnings on enjoyable activities or on the purchase of desired commodities.

Various kinds of tokens can be used in a reinforcement program—e.g., colored poker chips whose different colors represent different values, metal coins stamped to avoid counterfeiting, inexpensive foreign coins, paper tokens with different values printed on them, or credit cards (Lehrer, Schiff, and Kris, 1970) on which accumulated points can be tallied.

Different amounts of tokens can be earned contingent on the performance of distinct behaviors and the cost of preferred activities or commodities can vary. The activities or commodities that tokens can be exchanged for are called *back-up reinforcers*. Tokens become positive reinforcers (i.e., they increase the frequency of the behavior they follow) because the patient must have them in order to acquire the back-up reinforcers. Tokens, like money, become potent reinforcers because they allow the individual to buy the many things he personally desires. Having tokens is a necessary prerequisite to acquiring preferred activities and, therefore, tokens themselves become reinforcers.

Groups of patients in mental hospitals, in rehabilitation settings for delinquents, in institutions for the retarded, or children in public schools can be a part of a token reinforcement program. In the mental hospital, for example, the performance of various behaviors can be designated explicitly as worth a certain number of tokens. A sales-clerk assistant who assembles different commissary items may be allowed to earn three tokens for 30 minutes of work; or a ward cleaning assistant may be paid eight tokens for several hours of work that involves supplying different dormitories with cleaning equipment. Other jobs may include being a grooming assistant, a tour guide, a nursing assistant, or a dietary assistant; or the patient may be paid with tokens for engaging in specific self-care behaviors. These jobs and many more were part of Ayllon and Azrin's (1965) token reinforcement program for chronic mental patients. Tokens, therefore, can be made contingent on behaviors entailing vocational and housekeeping skills, involving social interaction and communication, relating to hygiene and grooming, and to many more; both off-ward and on-ward activities can be included in a token program. The tokens earned for the performance of these behaviors may be spent on activities, such as parties, home movies, watching T.V., field trips (Schaefer and Martin, 1969) or on such things as selected foods, cigarettes, extra privacy, better living quarters, and many other preferred reinforcers. A large supply of back-up reinforcers will be found if the patient's interests and activities are observed and are recorded. Anything that an individual enjoys doing or having can be made to function as a back-up reinforcer, which costs a certain amount of tokens.

With a token program, an environment can be created where adequate care is given to the patients but where adaptive and desirable behaviors—healthy behaviors—produce more than the usual amount of positive reinforcers. This environment will result in healtby activities being reinforced and becoming strong.

Nurses soon discover that the experience of working with patients on a token reinforcement program in a mental hospital is different from working with ones on a traditional ward. After the token reinforcement program begins to develop and the behaviors of the patient begin to change, many desirable "by-products" can be found. For instance, nurses will discover that they have more time to devote to activities other than the many custodial ones that consume much valuable time. Some of the beneficial results of a token reinforcement program at Patton State Mental Hospital are reported below by the change nurse. Her comments pertain to the program at the end of only one month. As she described:

> The project goes extremely well. We no longer have to call individuals for meals or coax them to go into the dining room. This used to require considerable time. Patients are taking the responsibility of getting to the dining room on time. It sometimes seems to us today that this came about automatically with the use of tokens. Other byproducts are that at mealtimes the general atmosphere seems more relaxed. There is no longer the mad rush to eat and get out. Patients get up without being called. Many of the patients we had to look out for in the beginning are now looking out for themselves. We hope this will continue. The night technician no longer has to go from bed to bed, calling the patients to get up for breakfast, get dressed for breakfast, and so on. She merely turns on the light and in three minutes goes back, and the patients who are up get their tokens. The ones who are not up get nothing. Very few are *not* up by then. . . . I have known some of the patients for five years, and for the first time I am seeing real progress made with them. I feel quite encouraged with our program, and we are learning as we go along. We understand fully now that we must reinforce good behavior when it occurs. Reinforcement is not as effective if it is given [too long] after the behavior has occurred. All the staff are extremely enthusiastic and feel that their own thinking is tremendously stimulated by what they are learning in this project.[1]

In sum, token reinforcement programs are useful for designing an environment that systematically and consistently strengthens the adaptive behaviors of patients. The basic ingredients of a token system are: (1) Explicitly designating desirable behaviors for the patients to engage in along with the number of tokens each behavior is worth. (2) Systematically reinforcing the occurrence of each behav-

---

[1]O. L. Gericke, "Practical use of operant conditioning procedures in a mental hospital," *Psychiatric Studies & Projects*, 3, 1965, 8–9.

ior that is designated; that is, administer tokens contingent on the occurrences of the target behaviors. (3) Providing a large variety of potent back-up reinforcers that can be exchanged for specific numbers or amounts of tokens. These back-up reinforcers are the preferred activities and commodities of the patients. To ascertain exactly what will function as back-up reinforcers, the nurse can interview and can observe the patients. The more back-up reinforcers available, the more likely tokens will be sought and, therefore, the greater the likelihood the patients will engage in the behaviors that earn tokens. (4) Establishing a system for recording each patient's progress, that is, record the occurrences of desirable behavior and the number of tokens earned, spent, and saved by each patient. Various recording procedures can be used.

Finally, it is important to mention that procedures useful in producing behavior (e.g., Shaping, Instructing, Demonstration–Imitation) as well as ones instrumental in increasing the complexity of behavior (e.g., Linking) can be employed in the token program to teach patients desired behaviors. In fact, all of the behavior modification procedures including those promoting durable changes in adaptive activities, such as social reinforcement, can be incorporated into the token reinforcement program.

Advantages and Disadvantages

There are several advantages of token programs. A carefully planned project can be instrumental in helping the patient to live more capably within the institution as well as in developing prerequisites for adjusting to the outside community.

Relatively large numbers of patients can be taught many important behaviors in a token-reinforcement program that focuses upon the needs and preferences of the individual. Such a program must designate behavior essential to the individual patient's welfare and back-up reinforcers that he personally desires.

The use of tokens to accelerate desirable behavior overcomes the disadvantages of exclusively employing primary reinforcers; that is, the individual patient will not readily become satiated with respect to tokens—tokens do not rapidly lose their reinforcing potency (tokens are not tied to only one condition of deprivation but instead are involved with the acquisition of *many different* types of back-up reinforcers). In addition, administering tokens contingent on behavior does not result in any interruption occurring because the reinforcer is consumed (tokens can be simply put into a pocket or purse).

Thus, tokens, which can become generalized-acquired reinforcers (see Chapter 3, Section 3.2), have advantages.

Tokens can be administered throughout the day immediately following designated target behaviors and then can be accumulated by the patient for the purchase of some potent back-up reinforcer at the end of the day. Therefore, the delay between the occurrence of the target behavior and the administration of the potent back-up reinforcer will be bridged by the token (Ayllon and Azrin, 1968). Tokens also can be saved up in a bank account. And tokens are portable, are not destroyed easily before they are cashed in, and are not duplicated readily (Ayllon and Azrin, 1968). Furthermore, tokens can be assigned different values so that the amount of reinforcement given to a patient can be adjusted easily to fit the quality or amount of his performances. Finally, a token provides a convenient index of the patient's progress in the hospital, which the nurse can record quickly.

The major disadvantage of a token system is that once the patient leaves it, he will come into touch with other kinds of reinforcers (e.g., social approval and disapproval), and unless they also are potent, the behavior changes which have resulted from the token program will dissipate. Token systems, however, can be instrumental in both strengthening important behaviors as well as in strengthening the patient's responsiveness to other kinds of reinforcers, so vital to long-term behavior changes (Sherman and Baer, 1969). Thus, tokens can be made progressively more intermittent, as the consequence of desirable behavior, with praise or other social reinforcers eventually supplanting them (e.g., Gericke, 1965).

The Individual Patient in the Token Reinforcement Program

As mentioned above, the personal preferences of the individual patient must be included in the token reinforcement program. In addition, it is necessary to implement specific behavior modification plans for patients who display bizarre or otherwise unadaptive behaviors. Thus, activities of the patient such as temper tantrums, incontinence, hallucinations, delusions, speaking inappropriately, incoherence, aggressive outbursts, eating problems, mutism, and so forth can be dealt with within the context of the token reinforcement program. Target behaviors for specific patients, therefore, can be defined, can be observed, can be recorded, and can be modified while the patient is a participating member of the program. Tokens, furthermore, can be employed in these individual projects as positive reinforcers administered contingent on the performance of certain desirable target behaviors and removed contingent on the performance of certain undesirable behaviors (Response-Cost).

Some patients may object initially to a token reinforcement program because they judge it to be arbitrary and unfair. Patients suddenly confronted with a change in the system, especially where new behaviors are required of them, may initially become defiant. But if a well-managed token program, which uses Positive Reinforcement procedures, allows each individual to profit from engaging in healthy behaviors and avoids punishing them for *not* performing these behaviors, the rebelliousness of the patients should be reduced (Bandura, 1969). Thus, as Bandura indicated, if the usual standards of the institution are maintained for all patients in terms of adequate food, living quarters, and so on, but better conditions (extra luxuries) are given to those patients who engage in the desirable behaviors, then each patient can decide for himself whether to practice them.

As a final comment in this section, it is important to mention that for some patients, notably for retarded children and adults, tokens initially may need to be coupled with the administration of primary or of other reinforcers in order for the tokens to take on reinforcing value. For many patients, however, verbal instructions about the token system will be all that is needed, and no direct teaching to use tokens for purchasing back-up reinforcers will be required.

TERMS AND QUESTIONS

Terms

Token reinforcement program
Back-up reinforcer

Questions

1. What are the basic ingredients of a token program?
2. What is the major disadvantage of a token program?
3. How can the severity of the reaction of mental patients to a token program be reduced?
4. How do you teach a child that tokens are valuable for him to acquire?

7.2 COMMUNITY-BASED REINFORCEMENT PROGRAMS

The Mental Patient and an Example of a Token Reinforcement Program Based in the Community

Token programs have been used in the education of public-school children (O'Leary and Drabman, 1971) and of retarded individuals (Birnbrauer et al., 1965) as well as of autistic children (Martin, 1969), in the rehabilitation of mental patients (Ayllon and Azrin, 1965), of delinquents, and recently in the activities of a Head Start Program (Miller and Schneider, 1970). Numerous token projects are currently in operation in various settings for many individuals with differing problems.

In Chapter 1, the feasibility of applying behavior modification procedures to groups of mentally disturbed patients was mentioned. Patients in traditional mental hospitals often deteriorate behaviorally to such an extent that they are unable to function capably in society, if released, even though the problems originally responsible for their hospitalization have diminished. Patients in the mental hospital are often forced into behaving passively and are not encouraged to make independent decisions; the smooth running of the ward often precludes treatment. Behavior deterioration, disculturation, and stigmatization characterize the long-term (chronic) mental patient. Unfortunately, the amount of time he spends in the hospital is often related to the development of his social breakdown (Honigfeld and Gillis, 1967) and not to his social repair.

The mental patient who spends years in the hospital, who has been abandoned by his family, who has been stigmatized by society, who has lost the requisite behaviors for capably living in society, who has developed "strange" mannerisms, who has become dependent or aggressive, apathetic, and withdrawn, and who no longer can make independent adaptive, decisions presents a grave problem. Treatment and attempts to prevent chronicity are possible with methods other than those customarily found in the traditional mental hospital. Behavior modification is one of these nontraditional methods.

Although behavior modification has not, as yet, provided definite answers to all the problems which beset the mental patient and which retard his rehabilitation, it has provided a promising strategy for discovering answers. The behavior modification approach to helping the psychologically disturbed individual recognizes that his environment is an extremely important factor in his rehabilitation. If the patient is placed in a mental hospital that does *not* specifically attempt to help him to develop and to maintain behaviors important to his successful re-adjustment in the outside community—that is, if the mental hospital does not create a suitable environment for the development of the patient's behaviors—long-term hospitalization (causing chronicity) is inevitable. The patient will spend the majority of his life in the mental hospital.

Rehabilitation must involve helping the mental patient to return to the community. The focus of rehabilitation, therefore, should be on accelerating behaviors necessary for adjustment in the community and should be on decelerating behaviors interfering with this adjustment. Consequently, activities that foster self-maintenance, interpersonal interaction, and gainful employment, should be accelerated and behaviors that are bizarre or strange should be decelerated (Paul, 1969). In addition, as Paul indicated, support for the patient in the community (e.g., by family or friends) should be provided once he is released from the hospital. These areas are targets for rehabilitation.

The following example represents one attempt to help mental patients to return to the outside society. As reported by Henderson and Scoles (1970),[2] their token reinforcement program is a community-based project for psychotic men. An overall objective appears to be the prevention of chronicity. The men (ages 18–55), called "residents" are housed in a facility known as Spruce House, which is located in the community. The staff at Spruce House regard the residents not as individuals who suffer from underlying mental diseases but as responsible people capable of altering their behaviors.

TARGET-BEHAVIOR AREAS. Essentially three areas are focused on to help the Spruce House residents to return to the outside community. They involve vocational skills, social skills, and individual behavior problems. In addition, there is a literacy program which is especially important to residents with educational deficiencies.

POSITIVE REINFORCERS. Token, social, and primary reinforcers are administered contingent on desirable behaviors. Tokens are exchangeable for preferred commodities and activities (e.g., candy, cigarettes, extra food, telephone calls, and passes). Residents who

---

[2]John D. Henderson and Pascal E. Scoles, Jr., "Conditioning techniques in a community-based operant environment for psychotic men," *Behavior Therapy*, 1, 1970, 245–251.

earn the most tokens each week are also entitled to select better living accommodations, preferred seating arrangements in the diningroom, and other privileges. Bonuses, in the form of prizes, may be administered to a patient contingent on his improving markedly from one week to the next. Bonus payments (tokens) also are available for maximum performances of target behaviors.

TOKENS ARE MADE CONTINGENT ON TARGET BEHAVIORS. Tokens can be earned for successfully performing the adaptive target behaviors. In the vocational program, the various jobs (e.g., "floorman," "laundryman," "headwaiter") are ranked according to the initiative and interpersonal skills required to perform them. Those positions that involve the greatest responsibility, independence, and social interaction on the part of the resident pay best. Thus, a resident can earn more tokens as a "headwaiter" (ranked high on the list) than as a "housekeeper" (ranked near the bottom of the list). Residents can be promoted to well-paying jobs contingent on a good performance of the job they are assigned. By reinforcing occupational skills as well as the qualities of initiative, responsibility, and social interaction, the authors are helping to bring these patients closer to living capably in the outside community.

Similarly, social activities (e.g., dances, athletics, field trips, discussion groups) are an important part of the treatment. Tokens can be earned for participating in these events. The degree of involvement in them, however, determines the number of tokens that can be earned. Thus, if a resident is involved only tangentially in an activity, he will earn fewer tokens than if he appears to be highly involved in it. The events can take place in the facility, both with and without volunteers from the community participating, or in the community itself. Token bonuses are given to residents who interact with individuals from the community. Because it is believed that this contact will help the patients to make the transition from Spruce House to the outside, it is reinforced.

Also, residents can earn tokens for showing a reduction in their behavior problems. Tokens are provided for achieving in the literacy program as well as for other improvements. For example, one resident who was deficient in communication skills was reinforced with tokens when he talked with others; an increase was found not only in his conversational behavior but in other desirable activities as well.

EVALUATION OF THE PROGRAM. By suspending reinforcers for a brief period of time and then reinstituting them, the authors demonstrated the immediate positive effects of the tokens on the social behaviors of the residents (see Chapter 5, Section 5.4 for a description of this reversal method of evaluation).

The long-term effects of the entire program were also evaluated. The results showed that there are fewer days of rehospitalization for the residents of Spruce House than for those of a City and a State hospital, although initial hospitalization for Spruce House individuals is somewhat longer. Also, graduates of Spruce House stay in the outside community and hold down jobs for more time, once released, than do patients released from the other two hospitals.

ADVANTAGES OF THE PROGRAM. The major advantages of this type of intensive program are its focus on returning the patient to the outside community and, in a related way, on preventing chronicity. To fulfill these constructive objectives, the patient's skills are developed during his stay within Spruce House; these skills are instrumental in helping him to maintain his residence in the society at large once he is released. Notably, the patient's behavior within the facility also is improved with this type of program. Furthermore, token reinforcement projects, such as the one conducted at Spruce House, often do not necessitate the presence of many staff members. According to the authors, only two or three on each shift were required for 20 residents. Another advantage of this reinforcement program, as the authors point out, is that the procedures and their influence on the individual patient are made explicit. This aspect enables the staff to decide upon necessary adjustments, as information is gathered, which are vital to each patient's treatment.

The Therapeutic Community

The prevention of chronicity[3] and the attempt to treat mental patients who have been inside the hospital for extended periods of time involves both helping them to *re-enter* the outside community and to *stay* there.

From the work of Paul (1969), Fairweather et al. (1969), Henderson and Scoles (1970), and others, two related topics that professionals must consider in attempting to rehabilitate mental patients are apparent. One concerns the treatment practices within the hos-

---

[3]Much of this section is based on Gordon L. Paul, "Chronic mental patient: Current status-future directions," *Psychological Bulletin*, 71, 1969, 81–94.

pital, and the other concerns the situations the patient encounters once he is in the community.

Within-hospital treatment practices, as already mentioned, should attempt to develop the patient's vocational, social, and educational skills as well as his independent decision making and responsibility. In addition, within-hospital treatment practices should attempt to reduce the patient's distressing behaviors that obviously would interfere with his being accepted and with his adjusting in the community. The goal of within-hospital treatment, in short, should be to help the patient to return to the outside society. Token reinforcement programs, which explicitly list behaviors essential for the patient to engage in (e.g., vocational, social, and educational), are useful in achieving the within-hospital objectives. The work of Henderson and Scoles (1970) exemplifies this approach, as does the effort of Atthowe and Krasner (1968), and others.

As Paul (1969) suggested, helping the patient to *stay* in the community involves teaching the patient and significant-others to live in "mutually supportive ways" both before the individual is released and through scheduled aftercare. The stresses that the patient encounters in the community during the first few months after he has left the hospital have a marked effect on the durability of his stay in the community. The patient and those who form a significant part of his daily environment must be helped to get along with one another and to handle the stresses which arise. Teaching family members and the patient in the home situation about drug administration and giving advice, encouragement, and reassurance has been found to prevent new hospitalizations; the instructor gradually can remove himself from the situation, while the family and the patient gradually assume control (Pasamanick, Scarpitti, and Dinitz, 1967).

Teaching the patient and the family members or additional significant-others to support one another can be instrumental in preventing both new hospitalization and rehospitalization for the patient. Employing behavior modification practices to *teach* and teaching behavior modification principles per se, which can help the patient and those individuals close to him to deal efficiently with signs of relapse or other problems, may be invaluable (see Chapter 3, Sections 3.5 and 3.6). The nurse may administer this function and then gradually may fade-out her participation, allowing the recipients of the instructions to gradually take over the job of supporting themselves.

Fairweather et al. (1969) have specifically attempted to remedy the problems associated with the patient's short postrelease stay in the community.[4] Basically, Fairweather and his colleagues have developed a community for mental patients in which the patients are able to maintain themselves with little professional contact.

The residents of this "community lodge" provide support for each other. They are primarily responsible for activities associated with running the facility (e.g., buying and preparing food), for helping each other with problems, and for operating a profitable business (i.e., a janitorial and community maintenance service). In short, they manage their own lives and make independent and responsible decisions with only a minimum of supervision. From the net profits of the business, the occupants are paid weekly salaries contingent on their contribution to the business and to the responsibilities in the lodge.

Prior to being sent to the lodge, the patients resided in the hospital setting. During their stay in the hospital, they were taught to make independent decisions and to exercise responsibility; the procedures used to teach them these vital activities were developed by Fairweather (1964). Briefly, groups of patients are formed who help each other improve. The patients in the group can earn reinforcers (money and passes) contingent on the level of initiative and responsibility they demonstrate. Reinforcers are administered by the group to which each patient belongs. The hospital staff reviews the adequacy of the various group decisions and can reinforce the group as a whole or can punish it. Although staff members participate in the group, the large majority of the decision-making activities take place without their recommendations during the daily group meetings. An important part of this decision-making teaching is the inclusion of a step system that requires progressively more initiative and responsibility from the patient. A group member receives money each week depending on his step level. And each advancement to a higher step requires more responsible behavior.

After this type of within-hospital education, the patients released to the community lodge are better prepared to meet the problems of managing themselves.

In the lodge, as in the hospital, the members learn to provide support for one another. Essentially, they become their own treatment experts and are able to function adequately in managing themselves. Follow-up information on effectiveness of the lodge is impressive. Its business is showing a profit, the residents are maintaining

---

[4] G. W. Fairweather, D. H. Sanders, H. Maynard, and D. L. Cressler, *Community Life for the Mentally Ill: An Alternative to Institutional Care* (Chicago, Illinois: Aldine Publishing Company, 1969).

employment and are, to say the least, more responsible than before for their own welfare. Staff participation in the ongoing activities of the lodge is minimal. In comparison to a similar group of patients receiving the same within-hospital treatment but who were subjected to traditional after-care procedures, the results of the community lodge project are very favorable.

A resident of the lodge can leave it, taking with him an increased ability to make decisions and to act responsibly. Many of the occupants, however, will not depart because they are without families and may have difficulty finding suitable employment; these individuals will profit much more from the lodge environment than from the hospital. In the lodge, they are part of a constructive and an independent group (Bandura, 1969).

QUESTIONS

1. What should be the target areas of within-hospital treatment for the mental patient?
2. What should after-care procedures involve for the mental patient?
3. How can behavior modification help to prevent chronicity among mental patients?

7.3 *A SYNTHESIS*

This chapter has dealt with the usefulness of the behavior modification approach to groups of individuals with mental problems. Central to the discussion was the description of token reinforcement programs which designate relevant activities for the patient to engage in (e.g., vocational behaviors and social activities); pay the patient with tokens contingent on his becoming involved in these behaviors; provide the patient with potent back-up reinforcers (extra luxuries, preferred activities) for which he can exchange his tokens. Although the focus of this chapter was on mental patients, the utility of the token system for other groups of people (e.g., retarded individuals and public school children) was noted.

Token reinforcement programs can improve the within-hospital functioning of the mental patient and, in addition, can provide him with important behaviors and behavior changes that will affect his readjustment in the community significantly. The work of Henderson and Scoles (1970), cited in this chapter, was discussed as one important within-hospital approach that utilized a token program for helping patients to re-enter the outside community. The work of Fairweather et al. (1969), which was also cited in this chapter, is not expressly a behavior modification approach but can be easily translated into behavior modification terminology (Davison, 1969). This method, which develops independence, initiative, and responsibility in mental patients while they are within the hospital setting and then transfers them to their own community environment, appears extremely promising for helping chronic mental patients.

Remaining cognizant that the patient is an individual—he has specific behavior problems and is responsive to particular back-up reinforcers—was stressed in this chapter as it has been in others. Furthermore, the necessity of viewing the mental patient not as a person plagued with psychological diseases, but rather as someone with behavior problems that prevent him from adjusting in the community was again mentioned. For the mental patient, it is also necessary to make his re-entry and durable stay in the outside community the overall objectives of treatment; these objectives are vital to eventuating his successful rehabilitation.

The environment in which a patient is treated and the environment to which he returns must foster the development of adaptive behaviors and the remediation of unadaptive ones. The significance of other people in the environment to which the patient returns and the nurse's role in teaching these other people as well as the patient behavior modification practices was mentioned again.

In the concluding statement (next), the discussion will once more focus on teaching the patient behavior modification principles —on teaching the patient self-control.

SUPPLEMENTARY READINGS

AYLLON, T., AND N. H. AZRIN *The Token Economy: A Motivational System for Therapy and Rehabilitation.* New York: Appleton-Century-Crofts, 1968.

FAIRWEATHER, G. W. *Methods for Experimental and Social Innovation.* New York: John Wiley & Sons, Inc., 1967.

———, D. H. Sanders, H. Maynard, and D. L. Cressler *Community Life for the Mentally Ill: An Alternative to Institutional Care.* Chicago: Aldine, 1969.

Lent, J. R., Judith LeBlanc, and J. E. Spradlin "Designing a Rehabilitative Culture for Moderately Retarded Adolescent Girls," in *Control of Human Behavior: From Cure to Prevention,* eds. R. Ulrich, T. Stachnik, and J. Mabry. Glenview, Illinois: Scott, Foresman and Company, 1970.

Phillips, E. L., Elaine A. Phillips, D. L. Fixsen, and M. M. Wolf "Achievement Place: Modification of the Behaviors of Pre-Delinquent Boys Within a Token Economy," *Journal of Applied Behavior Analysis,* 4, 1971, 45–59.

Schaefer, H. H., and P. L. Martin *Behavioral Therapy.* New York: McGraw-Hill Book Company, 1969.

eight Concluding Statement: The Development of Self-Control

A nurse can help a patient to modify his behavior by changing his environment in carefully planned ways. Thus, by administering positive reinforcers contingent on the performance of specifically designated desirable behavior, activity can be accelerated, and by withdrawing reinforcers, for example, contingent on the performance of undesirable behavior, activity can be decelerated. Behavior modification is a workable, humane, and meaningful approach to patient care. With this method, the skillful planning of the behavior modification program by a nurse, who is accurate and precise in her assessment of the patient's behavior and who is critical in her evaluation of the behavior modification program is essential—that is, the skillful, accurate, and precise management of the behavior modification program for the patient *by the nurse or by someone else who the nurse enlists* as a helping agent—is required. The nurse, the ward aides, the family, and others can be vital to an effective behavior modification program for the patient.

It is also possible and advantageous to educate a patient to help himself. The procedures that others use to modify a patient's behavior can be employed by the individual to modify his own behavior (Skinner, 1953). Patients who must reduce their intake of tobacco, food, alcohol, who should increase certain activities, such as studying assigned literature about health practices, or who should follow a prescribed diet, and so on can be taught to *control their environments and thereby to control their behaviors.* This competence is self-control.

All the various approaches that a patient can use to modify his own behavior and all the variables involved in learning self-control will not be reviewed here. For thorough examinations of this topic, please see other sources (e.g., Kanfer and Phillips, 1970; Cautela, 1969).

What will be advocated here involves an extension of the techniques and the procedures already discussed in this book; namely, educating the patient to become his own treatment expert (Goldiamond, 1965), which will entail teaching the patient how to assess his own behavior and the events that influence it, how to intervene by altering these events, and how to evaluate continually what he is doing. This type of guidance—self-help teaching—may be instrumental in both showing a patient how to improve his current behaviors and in arming him against the unbridled development of future difficulties.

Self-control can be instructed either by teaching the patient to apply certain procedures to particular problems or by teaching him about behavior modification principles *per se* as they relate to his own problems. The latter approach will allow the patient to formulate the procedures necessary for modifying his behavior (Goldiamond, 1965). This method is more general and may result in a greater understanding of the behavior modification principles so that the patient will be better able to *cope on his own* with future difficulties.

Teaching an individual behavior modification principles in order for him to be able to develop control over behavior he wishes to regulate is based on this assumption: part of the person's problem is due to his inability to analyze the relationship between his behavior and the controlling environmental events that precede and that follow his behavior (Kanfer et al., 1970). If the individual can be taught to recognize, to analyze, and to manipulate the occurrences that influence his behavior, he can learn to control it himself. To some extent, a person bothered by excesses in behavior (e.g., he overeats) or deficiencies in behavior (e.g., he does not study or does not exercise enough) fails to recognize exactly how events in his environment govern his behaviors. *Once the patient can learn to manipulate the conditions that control his activity, he can develop control over it himself.*

Thus, to teach an individual self-control, it is essential to teach him how he can identify the behavior he wants to regulate; determine the exact relationships between his activity and the crucial events affecting it; develop ways to alter these relationships and, thereby, promote self-control. When a patient can produce the behavior he wants when he wants it, he has achieved self-control. Consuming food each day at specifically designated times and in specifically designed ways and under specifically designated conditions in order to lose weight or to avoid obesity reflects self-control over eating behavior. Studying while at your desk and leaving it when you daydream or engage in any behavior not requiring intense thought and gradually increasing the time spent each day at your desk, eventually will result in good study habits (e.g., Goldiamond, 1965). This approach is one way of developing self-control over behavior.

Providing the patient with these essential teachings will involve instructing, demonstrating, practicing, and discussing the rudiments of behavior modification with him. The patient must learn to define accurately the behavior he wishes to change and the goals he has chosen for himself. In addition, he must learn to record precisely the situations that set the occasion for the activity he wishes to control as well as the events that reinforce it (its immediate and logical consequences).

If the problem involves excessive behavior (e.g., overeating), all the situations that set the occasion for overeating must be tallied. If the problem involves a deficient behavior (e.g., lack of exercise), all the situations that distract the individual from exercising must be listed clearly (e.g., phone ringing and interruptions from family).

The patient must learn to devise ways of altering the controlling effect of events on his behavior. The *actions* he takes in this regard are *self-controlling behaviors.* For example, eating only at specific times and in particular places without watching television are self-controlling behaviors for reducing the influence that many events (e.g., watching T.V.) have on eating. Developing this regulation is important for modifying obesity. [See Stuart's (1967) example below.] Thus, if watching T.V. or reading the newspaper set the occasion for consuming something, not allowing yourself to watch T.V. or to read when you eat (not engaging in any additional activity while you eat) will help to bring eating under the influence of more specific situations; that is, the control that numerous occasions have on eating will be narrowed to only a few. If the circumstances that influence a behavior can be narrowed to only a few relevant ones (e.g., eating only when you are at the diningroom table), the person will gain some control over the activity.

To foster the development of self-controlling behaviors, the individual should arrange his environment so that it will be favorable to their occurring. Thus, if overeating is to be regulated, the individual should keep food in the kitchen and not where it is openly in view, such as in the livingroom or in the bedroom. Obese people are likely to eat when they see food (Schacter, 1967). Similarly, if studying-behavior is to be increased, a sufficiently bright light, not a dim one, should be placed in the desk lamp (e.g., Goldiamond, 1965).

Strengthening the activity that a person must engage in for the purpose of developing self-control over a behavior requires reinforcement; that is, self-controlling behavior should be followed by reinforcers. Thus, during his beginning attempts, an individual can make the opportunity to engage in a highly reinforcing activity contingent on engaging in a self-controlling one. For example, the patient may decide to watch a certain amount of television (e.g., a favorite program) *only if* he has studied for a particular period of time; in effect, he makes a deal with himself whereby watching television becomes contingent on studying. By gradually increasing the time spent on the behavior to be accelerated (e.g., studying) or by gradually decreasing the behavior to be decelerated (e.g., eating), the individual will experience minimal discomfort and will maintain progress toward reaching his goals (Bandura, 1969).

One problem in strengthening self-controlling behaviors is that the occurrence of activity to be regulated can conflict with them; that is, the positive reinforcers which *immediately* follow the undesirable behavior—the behavior to be controlled—result in this behavior occurring frequently. And this effect can prevent self-control behaviors from developing.

For example, consider the problems the alcoholic has in maintaining sobriety, that is, self-control over excessive drinking. The positive reinforcers contingent on immoderate consumption of liquor are immediate. The positive reinforcers resulting from remaining temperate are delayed, although they are strong. Unfortunately, the smaller but more immediate reinforcers that follow the drinking can maintain this behavior and, thereby, can prevent the behaviors necessary for prolonged sobriety from occurring.

In other words, the immediate reinforcers contingent on some undesirable behaviors can exert more of a determining influence on the individual's current activities than the delayed reinforcers contingent on conflicting desirable behaviors (Whaley and Mallott, 1971). One of the major difficulties in treating some alcoholics may in fact be the following: The immediate positive reinforcers resulting from excessive drinking outweigh the delayed reinforcers resulting from prolonged sobriety. Sobriety will eventually lead to a better job, a happier home life, greater respect from significant-others, and so forth. Many alcoholics will agree to this assertion in group therapy and will maintain that they want the resultant events very much. But these strong reinforcers are delayed. The alcoholic must remain sober for an extended period before he can acquire them. The smaller reinforcers contingent on excessive drinking are more immediate and, because of this fact, the alcoholic may fail in treatment. Perhaps, if potent reinforcers were administered immediately following short periods of sobriety, that is, if self-controlling behaviors were reinforced immediately, the road to prolonged sobriety might be made smoother, and the goal of eventually controlling excessive drinking might be achieved.

Keeping daily records of progress (e.g., increments in study time or decrements in weight) will also yield reinforcers for self-controlling efforts. Continuous and up-to-date record keeping concerning the behavior to be regulated is an important element in acquiring self-control, not only because it reinforces self-controlling behaviors but also because it reminds the individual to continue to carry out the necessary procedures correctly (Bandura, 1969). Graphing behavior changes is a particularly useful way to make progress visible; patients should be instructed in this technique.

Other ways to strengthen self-controlling behaviors are available (e.g., Ferster, Nurnberger, and Levitt, 1962; Homme, 1965). Particularly helpful is to engage in a highly reinforcing substitute activity when the disposition to perform the undesirable behavior is great (e.g., taking a walk when the desire to eat between meals is strong).

The noticeable improvements that result from successful control over the target behavior, will eventually become potent reinforcers that maintain the continuation of the self-regulating efforts. Thus, when an individual can study, can exercise, or can eat appropriately for a long enough time to benefit from these activities, then explicit attempts to strengthen the self-controlling behaviors will no longer be necessary (Bandura, 1969; see Chapter 6, Section 6.2).

To illustrate the teaching of self-control, an example will be presented (Stuart, 1967)[1] in which eight obese women were taught to regulate their eating behaviors. Basically, Stuart taught these women to use procedures for altering their eating patterns and in-

---

[1]Richard B. Stuart, "Behavioral control of overeating," *Behaviour Research and Therapy*, 5, 1967, 357–365.

formed them of the rationale underlying these procedures. As part of the instruction, these women were taught to analyze their own behavior. To a large extent, self-control teaching equipped these women with methods for handling other problems in addition to obesity. Education about self-control may be a vital step toward preventative behavior modification.

The amount of time spent teaching these women was relatively short. The main sessions, in which assignments (prescriptions) were given, lasted approximately 30 minutes each (there were three sessions per week from four to five weeks). Other meetings were provided as needed. In addition, follow-up sessions were scheduled on a monthly basis for one year to evaluate the durability of behavior changes.

Although not presented to the patients in this specific order, Stuart's behavior prescriptions involved the following:

INSTRUCTING EACH PATIENT TO OBSERVE AND TO RECORD IMPORTANT INFORMATION RELATING TO HER PROBLEM. Information concerning the time and the quantity of food-and-drink consumption, for example, was recorded. The nature of the food ingested along with the circumstances under which eating occurred were included in this record. (The circumstances under which eating occurs [e.g., watching television] are important to identity because they set the occasion for consumption. As mentioned, the relationship between these antecedent events and the eating behavior can be changed, resulting in an alteration of the eating behavior.) Daily weight changes were also recorded. Each patient weighed herself at four designated times during the day, which provided the patient with clear information concerning the effect of food intake and reminded her of the program. In addition, each patient was asked to list reinforcing activities which she enjoyed performing as well as weight-related fears.

DEFINING THE GOALS EXPLICITLY. A one-to-two pound weight loss was designated as the weekly target of treatment. The long-term goal was the "stabilization of a reduced level of eating." A major concern in the early phases of the program was to increase the patient's control over the eating behavior *per se*, not to reduce her food intake. Decreasing what the patient ingested was very much a product of this self-control.

INSTRUCTING EACH PATIENT ABOUT PROCEDURES FOR EXERTING CONTROL OVER THE EATING BEHAVIOR ITSELF. One of these prescriptions required the patient to interrupt her eating for a brief period of time (2 to 3 minutes) by replacing her utensils on the table and by remaining seated. This assignment, which gradually was increased to five minutes, provided the patient with an early experience at self-control. In effect, this procedure showed her that eating is a behavior that can be broken down into components and gradually can be mastered. (This demonstration probably was reinforcing to the patient.) In another assignment, which was given later in treatment, the patient was told how to increase direct control over the eating behavior; that is, she was instructed to eat more slowly by placing only a small portion of food into her mouth and to replace her utensils on the table until she had swallowed. For an individual who has experienced relatively uncontrolled consumption, being able to control eating behavior directly in this fashion undoubtedly was a reinforcing experience—a self-control experience. Success at activities such as these strengthens future attempts at self-regulation.

Instructing Each Patient About Procedures for Exerting Control Over the Circumstances That Contribute to Unrestrained Eating. These assignments were intended to show the patient how to alter events that set the occasion for eating or that perhaps reinforce it. First, each patient was told to keep all food in the kitchen area, and most of this food would require preparation before eating; only one portion of a meal at a time would be prepared. This procedure acted to reduce "automatic" eating. By requiring that the patient go to the kitchen and to prepare the food, the author helped her to become alerted to impending eating. Second, the patient was told to make eating a "pure experience"; that is, each patient was instructed not to snack while engaging in any other pleasant activity, such as watching T.V. Thus, the control of events over consumption was narrowed (was lessened). The same instruction of making eating a pure experience would apply even if a person observes that events, such as watching T.V., do not precede ingestion but instead follow it. Thus, if watching T.V. is the usual consequence of going to open the refrigerator, eliminate this consequence (e.g., Goldiamond, 1965) in order to gain control over the eating behavior. Third, the patient was instructed to engage in some preferred activity at those times when the disposition to snack between meals was strong. Thus, between-meal eating, which to some extent time controls, was reduced by having a patient engage in some other reinforcing activity (e.g., telephoning a friend).[2] The disposition to consume, was to set

[2]Two patients who experienced problems in controlling their eating between meals were given an added treatment, namely, covert sensitization (see Cautela, 1969).

the occasion for some other reinforcing activity. Thus, if at 3:00 P.M. the patient had observed that she was likely to snack, she was instructed to call a friend. This substitute behavior as well as the mastery of self-control that it suggests are reinforcing to the patient. In addition, before engaging in this substitute behavior, the patient was to tell herself that she could regulate her snacking by performing alternative behaviors.

Stuart provided his patients with positive reinforcers for engaging in the self-controlling behavior. Thus, in addition to the reinforcement accruing from being able to regulate the problem, each patient was praised explicitly for her progress. During the teaching sessions, both discussions concerning recorded information and problems with prescriptions and discussions concerning new steps to be taken helped the patients to learn self-control. Throughout the meetings, the patients were encouraged to suggest relevant changes (e.g., substituting less fattening foods in their daily diet); their full participation in planning new steps was sought. By having the patients become involved in the treatment plan ("self-dosing"), the author facilitated their learning self-control.

Stuart reported that the patients not only were able to reduce overeating but also were able to stabilize their consumption at a reduced level. Thus, follow-up information (covering 52 weeks) indicated that the patients had made durable weight losses.

It is significant that several of the patients reported improvements in other behaviors. Notably, several of the women stated that they had extended self-control teaching to modify cigarette smoking and that they had been successful; in other words, a few patients had "self-applied" the procedures to another behavior problem and had altered it effectively.

In sum, Stuart was able to teach self-control behaviors to his patients by teaching them to analyze their own activity and to manipulate the important conditions affecting it. Also, he provided his patients with opportunities for reinforcement.

Self-control requires the full cooperation and participation of the person who wants to improve his behavior. To teach an individual effectively how to control his behavior requires that he understand the principles he is being taught and that he utilize them both for current problems and for ones yet to occur. Therefore, the individual who will profit most from being taught self-control, as described here, will probably be reasonably intelligent and will want to learn to regulate his behavior.

Expectant parents who have difficulty following necessary health-care practices; patients who are recuperating from various physical illnesses at home and who have problems in adhering to prescribed diets, taking medications, exercising, quitting smoking, and so on; out-patients from programs for alcoholics or drug users who must learn to control their addictions; and nursing students who need to learn to study more efficiently—all these could be candidates for self-control teaching. Any individual with a requisite amount of intelligence and motivation who has problems in controlling any one of his behaviors—because of a dearth of readily available procedures for managing his own environment—can be helped through self-control teaching. This approach can focus on the individual's present difficulties but should be complete enough to equip him with knowledge for self-applying behavior modification principles to his other current problems as well as to prevent future difficulties from getting out of control.

For too many patients, this type of important teaching (e.g., a large number of mental-hospital patients) may seem, at first glance, inapplicable. Although many mental hospital patients do possess the requisite intellectual skills to learn and to utilize self-control instruction, many do not possess the required motivation. Perhaps this problem may be handled by bringing these patients into touch with naturally occurring sources of reinforcement and by strengthening important adaptive behaviors. Goals such as these would be the precursors to effective self-control teaching. But to state exactly how the nurse can bring a mental-hospital patient to a level where he can profit from self-control instruction and thereby, can become his own treatment expert will, at present, be a formidable task—only one of the current challenges confronting those who attempt to help persons with behavior problems. Such challenges will stimulate the development of technologies for effectively and for meaningfully assisting individuals in behaving more capably.

Behavior modification provides an effective and a meaningful approach for meeting many of the responsibilities that currently confront nurses. To this writer, it appears that the progressive refinement and the further extension of behavior modification in nursing will result in its continuing to be of value to nurses as their roles develop in the future.

SUPPLEMENTARY READINGS

Ferster, C. B., J. I. Nurnberger, and E. B. Levitt "The Control of Eating," *Journal of Mathetics*, 1, 1962, 87–109.

GOLDIAMOND, I. "Self Control Procedures in Personal Behavior Problems," *Psychological Reports*, 17, 1965, 851–868.

HOMME, L. E. "Perspectives in Psychology—XXIV: Control of Coverants, the Operants of the Mind," *Psychological Record*, 15, 1965, 501–511.

STUART, R. B. "A Three-Dimensional Program for the Treatment of Obesity," *Behaviour Research and Therapy*, 9, 1971, 177–186.

———, AND B. DAVIS *Slim Chance in a Fat World: Behavioral Control of Obesity*. Champaign, Ill.: Research Press Company, 1972.

References

ABRAMSON, E. E., AND RICHARD A. WUNDERLICH "Dental Hygiene Training for Retardates: An Application of Behavioral Techniques." Paper presented at the meeting of the Eastern Psychological Association, Atlantic City, New Jersey, 1970.

ACKER, L., W. R. KELLEY, C. R. MASON, AND D. M. MCAMMOND "Short-Term Behavior Modification for Speech in a Young Boy." Paper presented at the Canadian Psychological Association, Winnipeg, Canada, 1970.

ADDISON, R. M., AND L. HOMME "The Reinforcing Event (RE) Menu," *NSPI Journal*, 5, No. 1, 1966, 8–9.

AIKEN, LINDA H. "Patient Problems Are Problems in Learning," *American Journal of Nursing*, 70, No. 9, 1970, 1916–1918.

ALLEN, K. EILEEN, AND FLORENCE R. HARRIS "Elimination of a Child's Excessive Scratching by Training the Mother in Reinforcement Procedures," *Behaviour Research and Therapy*, 4, 1966, 79–84.

ARADINE, CAROLYN R., AND MARC F. HANSEN "Nursing in a Primary Health Care Setting," *Nursing Outlook*, 18, 1970, 45–46.

ATTHOWE, J., AND L. KRASNER "Preliminary Report on the Application of Contingent Reinforcement Procedures (Token Economy) on a 'Chronic' Psychiatric Ward," *Journal of Abnormal Psychology*, 73, No. 1, 1968, 37–43.

AYLLON, T. "Intensive Treatment of Psychotic Behaviour by Stimulus Satiation and Food Reinforcement," *Behaviour Research and Therapy*, 1, 1963, 53–61.

———, AND N. H. AZRIN "The Measurement and Reinforcement of Behavior of Psychotics," *Journal of the Experimental Analysis of Behavior*, 8, 1965, 357–383.

——— *The Token Economy: A Motivational System for Therapy and Rehabilitation*. New York: Appleton-Century-Crofts, 1968.

AYLLON, T., AND E. HAUGHTON "Modification of Symptomatic Verbal Behaviour of Mental Patients," *Behaviour Research and Therapy*, 2, 1964, 87–97.

AYLLON, T., AND J. MICHAEL "The Psychiatric Nurse as a Behavioral Engineer," *Journal of the Experimental Analysis of Behavior*, 2, 1959, 323–334.

AZRIN, N. H., AND J. POWELL "Behavioral Engineering: The Use of Response Priming to Improve Prescribed Self-Medication," *Journal of Applied Behavior Analysis*, 2, 1969, 39–42.

AZRIN, N. H., H. RUBIN, F. O'BRIEN, T. AYLLON, AND D. ROLL "Behavioral Engineering: Postural Control by a Portable-Operant Apparatus," *Journal of Applied Behavior Analysis*, 1, 1968, 99–108.

BACHRACH, A. J., W. J. ERWIN, AND J. P. MOHR "The Control of Eating Behavior in an Anorexic By Operant Conditioning Techniques," in *Case Studies in Behavior Modification*, eds. L. P. Ullmann and L. Krasner. New York: Holt, Rinehart & Winston, Inc., 1965.

BAER, D. M. "A Case for the Selective Reinforcement of Punishment," in *Behavior Modification in Clinical Psychology*, eds. C. Neuringer and J. L. Michael. New York: Appleton-Century-Crofts, 1970.

———, R. F. PETERSON, AND J. A. SHERMAN "Building an Imitative Repertoire by Programming Similarity between Child and Model as Discriminative for Reinforcement." Paper read at the biennial meeting of the Society for Research in Child Development, Minneapolis, Minnesota, 1965.

BAER, D. M., AND MONTROSE M. WOLF "The Entry into Natural Communities of Reinforcement." Paper presented at the meeting of the American Psychological Association, Washington, D.C., 1967.

———, AND T. R. RISLEY Some Current Dimensions of Applied Behavior Analysis," *Journal of Applied Behavior Analysis*, 1, 1968, 91–97.

BALL, T. S. "Issues and Implications of Operant Conditioning: The Re-establishment of Social Behavior," *Hospital & Community Psychiatry*, 19, 1968, 230–232.

BANDURA, A. *Principles of Behavior Modification*. New York: Holt, Rinehart & Winston, Inc., 1969.

BARRETT, BEATRICE H. "Reduction in Rate of Multiple Tics by Free Operant Conditioning Methods," *Journal of Nervous and Mental Disease*, 135, 1962, 187–195.

BARTON, ELIZABETH S., D. GUESS, E. GARCIA, AND D. M. BAER "Improvement of Retardates' Mealtime Behaviors by Timeout Procedures Using Multiple Baseline Techniques," *Journal of Applied Behavior Analysis*, 3, 1970, 77–84.

BERGIN, A. E. "The Evaluation of Therapeutic Outcomes," in *Handbook of Psychotherapy and Behavior Change,* eds. A. E. Bergin and S. L. Garfield. New York: John Wiley & Sons, Inc., 1971.

BERKOWITZ, S., P. SHERRY, AND BARBARA A. DAVIS "Teaching Self-Feeding Skills to Profound Retardates Using Reinforcement and Fading Procedures," *Behavior Therapy,* 2, 1971, 62–67.

BERNAL, M., J. DURYEE, H. PRUETT, AND B. BURNS "Behavior Modification and the Brat Syndrome," *Journal of Consulting and Clinical Psychology,* 32, 1968, 447–455.

BIJOU, S. W. "Implications of Behavioral Science for Counseling and Guidance." Paper presented at the Cubberly Conference, Stanford University, Stanford, California, July, 1965.

________, AND D. M. BAER *Child Development I: A Systematic and Empirical Theory.* New York: Appleton-Century-Crofts, 1961.

BIJOU, S. W., R. F. PETERSON, AND M. H. AULT "A Method to Integrate Descriptive and Experimental Field Studies at the Level of Data and Empirical Concepts," *Journal of Applied Behavior Analysis,* 1, 1968, 175–191.

BIRNBAUER, J. S., M. M. WOLF, J. D. KIDDER, AND C. E. TAUGE "Classroom Behavior of Retarded Pupils with Token Reinforcement," *Journal of Experimental Child Psychology,* 2, 1965, 219–235.

BLACKHAM, G. J., AND A. SILBERMAN *Modification of Child Behavior.* Belmont, California: Wadsworth Publishing Company, Inc., 1971.

BROWNING, R. M., AND D. O. STOVER *Behavior Modification in Child Treatment: An Experimental and Clinical Approach.* New York: Aldine-Atherton, 1971.

CAHOON, D. D. "Issues and Implications of Operant Conditioning: Balancing Procedures Against Outcomes," *Hospital & Community Psychiatry,* 19, 1968, 228–229.

CAUTELA, J. R. "Behavior Therapy and Self-Control: Techniques and Implications," in *Behavior Therapy: Appraisal and Status,* ed. C. M. Franks. New York: McGraw-Hill Book Company, 1969.

COE, W. C. "A Family Operant Program." Paper presented at the meeting of the Western Psychological Association, Los Angeles, Calif., 1970.

CONGER, J. C. "The Treatment of Encopresis by the Management of Social Consequences," *Behavior Therapy,* 1, 1970, 386–390.

DAVIS, ELLEN D. "Give a Bath," *American Journal of Nursing,* 70, No. 11, 1970, 2366–2367.

DAVISON, G. C. "Appraisal of Behavior Modification Techniques with Adults in Institutional Settings," in *Behavior Therapy: Appraisal and Status,* ed. C. M. Franks. New York: McGraw-Hill Book Company, 1969.

ENGELN, R., J. KNUTSON, L. LAUGHY, AND W. GARLINGTON "Behavior Modification Techniques Applied to a Family Unit—A Case Study," *Journal of Child Psychology and Psychiatry,* 9, 1968, 245–252.

FAIRWEATHER, G. W. (ed.) *Social Psychology in Treating Mental Illness: Experimental Approach.* New York: John Wiley & Sons, Inc., 1964.

———, D. H. SANDERS, H. MAYNARD, AND D. L. CRESSLER *Community Life for the Mentally Ill: An Alternative to Institutional Care.* Chicago, Illinois: Aldine Publishing Company, 1969.

FERSTER, C. B., J. I. NURNBERGER AND E. B. LEVITT "The Control of Eating," *Journal of Mathetics,* 1, 1962, 87–110.

FERSTER, C. B., AND MARY C. PERROTT *Behavior Principles,* New York: Appleton-Century-Crofts, 1968.

FORDYCE, W., R. S. FOWLER, J. F. LEHMANN, AND BARBARA J. DELATEUR "Some Implications of Learning in Problems of Chronic Pain," *Journal of Chronic Diseases,* 21, 1968, 179–190.

FREDLUND, DELPHIE "Juevenile Delinquency and School Nursing," *Nursing Outlook,* 18, No. 5, 1970, 57–59.

GAMBRILL, E. D., E. J. THOMAS, AND R. D. CARTER "Procedure for Socio-Behavioral Practice in Open Settings," in *Utilization and Appraisal of Socio-Behavioral Techniques in Social Welfare,* eds. E. J. Thomas, R. D. Carter, and E. D. Gambrill. Michigan: Office of Research Administrations, The University of Michigan School of Social Work, Ann Arbor, Mich., June, 1970.

GERICKE, O. L. "Practical Use of Operant Conditioning Procedures in a Mental Hospital," *Psychiatric Studies & Projects,* 3, 1965, 2–10.

GODA, S. "Speech Development in Children," *American Journal of Nursing,* 70, No. 2, 1970, 276–278.

GOFFMAN, E. *Asylums.* New York: Doubleday, 1961.

GOLDIAMOND, I. "Self-Control Procedures in Personal Behavior Problems," *Psychological Reports,* 17, 1965, 851–868.

GOODKIN, R. "Case Studies in Behavioral Research in Rehabilitation," *Perceptual and Motor Skills,* 23, 1966, 171–182.

HAHN, ANNE, AND NANCY DOLAN "After Coronary Care—Then What?" *American Journal of Nursing,* 70, No. 11, 1970, 2350–2352.

HALL, R. V. *Behavior Management Series—Part I. Behavior Modification: The Measurement of Behavior.* Merriam, Kansas: H&H Enterprises, Inc., 1970.

———, AND MARCIA BRODEN Behavior Changes in Brain-Injured Children Through Social Reinforcement," *Journal of Experimental Child Psychology,* 5, 1967, 463–479.

HARRIS, F. R., M. K. JOHNSTON, C. S. KELLEY, AND M. M. WOLF "Effects of Positive Social Reinforcement on Regressed Crawling of a Nursery School Child," *Journal of Educational Psychology,* 55, 1964, 35–41.

HAWKINS, R., R. PETERSON, EDDA SCHWEID, AND S. BIJOU "Behavior Therapy in the Home: Amelioration of Problem Parent-Child Relations with the Parent in the Therapeutic Role," *Journal of Experimental Child Psychology,* 4, 1966, 99–107.

HECHT, AMY B. "Self-Medication, Inaccuracy, and What Can Be Done," *Nursing Outlook,* 18, 1970, 30–31.

HENDERSON, J. D., AND P. E. SCOLES, JR. "Conditioning Techniques in a Community-Based Operant Environment for Psychotic Men," *Behavior Therapy*, 1, 1970, 245–251.

HOLLAND, C. J. "Elimination by the Parents of Fire-setting Behaviour in a 7-year-old boy," *Behaviour Research and Therapy*, 7, 1969, 135–137.

HOMME, L. E. "Perspectives in Psychology—XXIV: Control of Coverants, the Operants of the Mind," *Psychological Record*, 15, 1965, 501–511.

________, A. P. CSANYI, MARY A. GONZALES, AND JAMES R. RECHS *How to Use Contingency Contracting in the Classroom*. Champaign, Illinois: Research Press, 1971.

HOMME, L. E., P. C. DEBACA, J. V. DEVINE, R. STEINHORST, AND E. J. RICKERT "Use of the Premack Principle in Controlling the Behavior of Nursery School Children," *Journal of the Experimental Analysis of Behavior*, 6, 1963, 544.

HONIGFELD, G., AND R. GILLIS "The Role of Institutionalization in the Natural History of Schizophrenia," *Diseases of the Nervous System*, 28, 1967, 660–663.

HOPKINS, B. L. "Effects of Candy and Social Reinforcement, Instructions, and Reinforcement Schedule Leaning on the Modification and Maintenance of Smiling," *Journal of Applied Behavior Analysis*, 1, 1968, 121–129.

ISAACS, W., J. THOMAS, AND I. GOLDIAMOND "Application of Operant Conditioning to Reinstate Verbal Behavior in Psychotics," *Journal of Speech and Hearing Disorders*, 25, 1960, 8–12.

JONES, MARY C. "The Elimination of Children's Fears," *Journal of Experimental Psychology*, 7, 1924, 382–390.

KANFER, F. H., AND JEANNE S. PHILLIPS *Learning Foundations of Behavior Therapy*. New York: John Wiley & Sons, Inc., 1970.

KENNEDY, TRUDY "Treatment of Chronic Schizophrenia by Behaviour Therapy: Case Reports," *Behaviour Research and Therapy*, 2, 1964, 1–6.

KRASNER, L. "The Operant Approach in Behavior Therapy," in *Handbook of Psychotherapy and Behavior Change*, eds. A. E. Bergin and S. L. Garfield. New York: John Wiley & Sons, Inc., 1971.

LEBOW, M. D. "Behavior Modification for the Family," in *Family Therapy: An Introduction to Theory and Technique*, eds. G. Erickson and T. Hogan. Belmont, California: Brooks/Cole, 1972.

________, S. GELFAND, AND W. R. DOBSON "The Aversive conditioning of a Phenothiazine-Induced Respiratory Stridor," *Behavior Therapy*, 1, 1970, 222–227.

LEHRER, P., L. SCHIFF AND A. KRIS "The Use of a Credit Card in a Token Economy," *Journal of Applied Behavior Analysis*, 3, 1970, 289–291.

LEITENBERG, H., W. STEWART AGRAS, AND L. THOMSON "A Sequential Analysis of the Effect of Selective Positive Reinforcement in Modifying Anorexia Nervosa," *Behaviour Research and Therapy*, 6, 1968, 211–218.

LEROUX, ROSE, AND DONNA ARLTON "The Foster Grandparent Program," *Nursing Forum*, 8, No. 4, 1969, 405–415.

LOVAAS, O. I. "A Behavioral Approach to the Treatment of Childhood Schizophrenia," in *Minnesota Symposia on Child Psychology*, Vol. 1, ed. J. T. Hill. Minneapolis: University of Minnesota Press, 1967.

———, J. P. BERBERICH, B. F. PERLOFF, AND B. SCHAEFFER "Acquisition of Imitative Speech by Schizophrenic Children," *Science*, 151, 1966, 705–707.

LOVAAS, O. I., G. FREITAG, VIVIAN J. GOLD, AND IRENE C. KASSORLA "Experimental Studies in Childhood Schizophrenia: Analysis of Self-Destructive Behavior," *Journal of Experimental Child Psychology*, 2, 1965, 67–84.

LOVAAS, O. I., G. FREITAG, M. KINDER, B. RUBENSTEIN, B. SCHAEFFER, AND J. Q. SIMMONS "Establishment of Social Reinforcers in Two Schizophrenic Children on the Basis of Food," *Journal of Experimental Child Psychology*, 4, 1966, 109–125.

LOVAAS, O. I., B. SCHAEFFER, AND J. Q. SIMMONS "Building Social Behavior in Autistic Children by Use of Electric Shock," *Journal of Experimental Research In Personality*, 1, 1965, 99–109.

LOVAAS, O. I., AND J. Q. SIMMONS "Manipulation of Self-Destruction in Three Retarded Children," *Journal of Applied Behavior Analysis*, 2, 1969, 143–157.

LOYND, JENNI, AND A. BARCLAY "A Case Study in Developing Ambulation in a Profoundly Retarded Child," *Behaviour Research and Therapy*, 8, 1970, 207.

MADSEN, C. H., JR. "Positive Reinforcement in the Toilet Training of a Normal Child: A Case Report," in *Case Studies in Behavior Modification*, eds. L. P. Ullmann and L. Krasner. New York: Holt, Rinehart & Winston, Inc., 1965.

MANN, R. A. "The Use of Contingency Contracting to Control Obesity in Adult Subjects." Paper presented at the Western Psychological Association, San Francisco, Calif., 1971.

MARTIN, G. L. "Operant Conditioning at the Manitoba School: A Description of Program Development," *The Manitoba School (MS) Journal*, 1, 1969, 11–17.

MEHRABIAN, A. *Tactics of Social Influence*. Englewood Cliffs, N.J.: Prentice-Hall, Inc., 1970.

MERENESS, DOROTHY, AND LOUIS J. KARNOSH *Essentials of Psychiatric Nursing*. St. Louis: The C. V. Mosby Company, 1966.

MILBY, J. B. "Modification of Extreme Social Isolation by Contingent Social Reinforcement," *Journal of Applied Behavior Analysis*, 3, 1970, 149–152.

MILLER, H. R., MARY E. PATTON, AND K. R. HENTON "Behavior Modification in a Profoundly Retarded Child: A Case Report," *Behavior Therapy*, 2, 1971, 375–384.

MILLER, L. K. AND O. L. MILLER "Reinforcing Self-Help Group Activities of Welfare Recipients," *Journal of Applied Behavior Analysis*, 3, 1970, 57–64

MILLER, L. K., AND R. SCHNEIDER "The Use of a Token System in Project Head Start," *Journal of Applied Behavior Analysis*, 3, 1970, 213–220.

O'LEARY, K. D., AND R. DRABMAN "Token Reinforcement Programs in the Classrooms: A Review," *Psychological Bulletin*, 75, 1971, 379–398.

O'LEARY, K. D., S. O'LEARY, AND W. C. BECKER "Modification of a Deviant Sibling Interaction Pattern in the Home," *Behaviour Research and Therapy*, 5, 1967, 113–120.

OSBORNE, J. GRAYSON "Free-Time as a Reinforcer in the Management of Classroom Behavior," *Journal of Applied Behavior Analysis*, 2, 1969, 113–118.

PASAMANICK, B., F. R. SCARPITTI, AND S. DINITZ *Schizophrenics in the Community*. New York: Appleton-Century-Crofts, 1967.

PATTERSON, G. R., AND M. E. GUILLON *Living with Children: New Methods for Parents and Teachers*. Champaign, Illinois: Research Press, 1968.

PATTERSON, G. R., S. MCNEAL, N. HAWKINS, AND R. PHELPS "Reprogramming the Social Environment," *Journal of Child Psychology and Psychiatry*, 8, 1967, 181–195.

PATTERSON, G. R., R. S. RAY, AND D. A. SHAW "Direct Intervention in Families of Deviant Children," *Oregon Research Institute Bulletin*, 8, No. 9, 1968.

PAUL, G. L. "Chronic Mental Patient: Current Status-Future Directions," *Psychological Bulletin*, 71, 1969, 81–94.

PREMACK, D. "Prediction of the Comparative Reinforcement Values of Running and Drinking," *Science*, 139, 1963, 1062–1063.

PUTT, ARLENE M. "One Experiment in Nursing Adults with Peptic Ulcers," *Nursing Research*, 19, No. 6, 1970, 484–494.

REESE, ELLEN P. *The Analysis of Human Operant Behavior*. Dubuque: Wm. C. Brown Company, Publishers, 1966.

REMILLET, JUNE, AND SADIE READING "Adapting to Changing Community Health Needs," *Nursing Outlook*, 18, No. 10, 1970, 47–49.

REYNOLDS, G. S. *A Primer of Operant Conditioning*. Glenview, Illinois: Scott, Foresman and Company, 1968.

RICE, H. K., MARTHA W. MCDANIEL, AND SARAH L. DENNEY "Operant Conditioning Techniques for Use in the Physical Rehabilitation of the Multiply Handicapped Retarded Patient," *Physical Therapy*, 48, No. 4, 1968, 342–346.

RISLEY, T. R. "Behavior Modification: An Experimental-Therapeutic Endeavor," in *Behavior Modification and Ideal Mental Health Services*, eds. L. A. Hamerlynck, P. O. Davidson, and L. E. Acker. Calgary, Alberta, Canada: University of Calgary, 1969.

SCHACTER, S. "Cognitive Effects on Bodily Functioning: Studies of Obesity and Eating," in *Neurophysiology and Emotion*, ed. D. C. Glass. New York: Rockefeller University Press and Russell Sage Foundation, 1967.

SCHAEFER, H. H., AND P. L. MARTIN "Behavioral Therapy for 'Apathy' of Hospitalized Schizophrenics," *Psychological Reports*, 19, 1966, 1147–1158.

——— *Behavioral Therapy*. New York: McGraw-Hill Book Company, 1969.

SECOR, SOPHIA M. "Colostomy Rehabilitation," *American Journal of Nursing*, 70, No. 11, 1970, 2400–2401.

SHANNON, IRIS R. "More Nursing per Square Mile," *Nursing Outlook*, 18, 1970, 42–44.

SHERMAN, J. A. "Use of Reinforcement and Imitation to Reinstate Verbal Behavior in Mute Psychotics," *Journal of Abnormal Psychology*, 70, 1965, 155–164.

———, AND D. M. BAER "Appraisal of Operant Therapy Techniques with Children and Adults," in *Behavior Therapy: Appraisal and Status*, ed. C. M. Franks. New York: McGraw-Hill Book Company, 1969.

SKINNER, B. F. *Science and Human Behavior*. New York: The Macmillan Company, 1953.

STUART, R. B. "Behavioral Control of Overeating," *Behaviour Research and Therapy*, 5, 1967, 357–365.

——— "Operant-Interpersonal Treatment for Marital Discord," *Journal of Consulting and Clinical Psychology*, 33, 1969, 675–682.

——— *Trick or Treatment: How and When Psychotherapy Fails*. Champaign, Illinois: Research Press, 1970.

TATE, B. G., AND GEORGE S. BAROFF "Aversive Control of Self-Injurious Behavior in a Psychotic Boy," *Behaviour Research and Therapy*, 4, 1966, 281–287.

TAYLOR, JOSEPHINE, AND CHARLES M. GAITZ "Obstacles Encountered in the Rehabilitation of Geriatric Patients," *Nursing Forum*, 8, No. 1, 1969, 64–73.

TREFFRY, D., G. L. MARTIN, G. SAMELS, AND C. WATSON "Operant Conditioning of Grooming Behavior in Severely Retarded Girls," *Mental Retardation*, 8, No. 4, 1970, 29–33.

TROMBLY, CATHERINE A. "Principles of Operant Conditioning Related to Orthotic Training of Quadriplegic Patients," *The American Journal of Occupational Therapy*, 20, No. 5, 1966, 217–220.

TUDOR, LEA L. "Bladder and Bowel Retraining," *American Journal of Nursing*, 70, No. 11, 1970, 2391–2393.

TURNER, RUBY "A Method of Working with Disturbed Children," *American Journal of Nursing*, 70, No. 10, 1970, 2146–2151.

"Two Days of Everyweek," *American Journal of Nursing*, 70, No. 1, 1970, 77.

ULLMANN, L. P., AND L. KRASNER *A Psychological Approach to Abnormal Behavior*. Englewood Cliffs, N.J.: Prentice-Hall, Inc., 1969.

——— (eds.) *Case Studies in Behavior Modification*. New York: Holt, Rinehart & Winston, Inc., 1965.

VALENTINE, LOIS R. "Self-Care Through Group Learning," *American Journal of Nursing*, 70, No. 10, 1970, 2140–2142.

WAHLER, R. G. "Behavior Therapy for Oppositional Children: Love Is Not Enough." Paper presented at the annual meeting of the Eastern Psychological Association, Washington, D.C., 1968.

WAHLER, R. G. "Oppositional Children: A Quest for Parental Reinforcement Control," *Journal of Applied Behavior Analysis*, 2, 1969, 159–170.

———, G. H. WINKEL, R. F. PETERSON, AND D. C. MORRISON "Mothers as Behavior Therapists for Their Own Child," *Behaviour Research and Therapy*, 3, 1965, 113–134.

WATSON, J. B., AND ROSALIE RAYNOR "Conditioned Emotional Reactions," *Journal of Experimental Psychology*, 3, 1920, 1–14.

WHALEY, D. L., AND R. W. MALOTT *Elementary Principles of Behavior*. New York: Appleton-Century-Crofts, 1971.

WILLIAMS, C. D. "The Elimination of Tantrum Behavior by Extinction Procedures: Case Report," *Journal of Abnormal and Social Psychology*, 59, 1959, 269.

WOLF, M. M., JAY S. BIRNBRAUER, TOM WILLIAMS, AND JULIA LAWLER "A Note on Apparent Extinction of the Vomiting Behavior of a Retarded Child," in *Case Studies in Behavior Modification*, eds. L. P. Ullmann and L. Krasner. New York: Holt, Rinehart & Winston, Inc., 1965.

WOLPE, J., AND A. A. LAZARUS *Behavior Therapy Techniques*. New York: Pergamon Press, 1966.

YATES, A. J. "Symptoms and Symptom Substitution," *Psychological Review*, 65, 1958, 371–374.

ZEILBERGER, JANE, SUE E. SAMPEN, AND H. N. SLOANE, JR. "Modification of a Child's Problem Behaviors in the Home with the Mother as Therapist," *Journal of Applied Behavior Analysis*, 1, 1968, 47–53.

Index

A

Abramson, A. A., 95
Accelerating desirable behavior (*see* Negative Reinforcement procedure; Positive Reinforcement procedure; Stimuli)
Accelerating effect of stimuli, 39–40
Acker, L., 45, 207
Acquired reinforcers, 50–53, 131
Activity (personalized) reinforcers, 55–57, 131
  case study, 61–63
Addison, R. M., 61
Agras, W. Stewart, 213
Aiken, Linda H., 8, 17, 18, 109, 119–120
Allen, K. Eileen, 103, 105
Anorexia nervosa, 213–215
Anxiety, 15–18
  systematic desensitization, 17
Apathy, 211–213
Aradine, Carolyn R., 109
Arlton, Donna, 116
Assessment, 11, 18–19, 22, 175
  baseline information, 182–185
  defining behavior, 176–177
  observing behavior, 178–181
  recording behavior, 179–181, 185 198
    frequency of activities, 186
    graphing, 192–194
    interval recording, 186–189
    time sampling, 189–191
Atthowe, J., 240
Ault, M. H., 178
Aversive Stimulation procedure, 127, 137–142, 147, 154, 156, 166, 181, 204
  case study, 139–141
  compared to Extinction, 159–160
  compared to Withdrawal of Positive Reinforcement, 158–159
Ayllon, T., 20, 51, 150, 157–158, 161, 163, 167, 231, 234, 236
Azrin, N. H., 20, 51, 128, 231, 234, 236

B

Bachrach, A. J., 213
Baer, D. M., 12, 18, 44, 79, 97, 122–123, 130, 139, 207, 234
Ball, T. S., 26
Bandura, A., 25, 31, 42, 78, 139, 153, 235, 242, 248, 249
Barclay, A., 216
Baroff, George S., 139
Barrett, Beatrice A., 146
Barton, Elizabeth S., 220
Baseline information, 182–185
Becker, W. C., 177
Behavioral contract, 62–63, 173
Behavioral engineering, 128–129
Behavior deterioration, 19–20
Berberich, J. P., 76
Bergin, A. E., 4
Berkowitz, S., 82
Bernal, M., 126
Bijou, S. W., 18, 44, 178, 201
Birnbrauer, J. S., 236
Blackham, G. J., 184
Bribery, 28–29, 62
Broden, Marcia, 217–218
Browning, R. M., 9

C

Cahoon, D. D., 27
Carter, R. D., 32
Cautela, J. R., 246
Chaining, 86
Chronic pain, 222–225
Classical conditioning (*see* Respondent conditioning)
Coe, W. C., 62
Communities of reinforcement, 122–123
Community-based reinforcement programs, 236–242
  therapeutic community, 239–242
Conditional stimulus, 15
Conger, J. C., 113–114
Contingent relationship, 41–42 (*see also* Decelerating undesirable behavior; Negative Reinforcement procedure; Positive Reinforcement procedure)
Continuous reinforcement schedule, 65
Control, 29–31, 35
Conventional line graph, 192–194

D

Davis, Barbara A., 82
Davis, Ellen D., 52
Davison, G. C., 243
Decelerating effect of stimuli, 40
Decelerating undesirable behavior, 135–174
  Aversive Stimulation, 137–142, 158–160, 171
  Extinction, 152–161, 171–172
  Reinforcing Other Behavior, 162–165, 171
  Satiation, 148–152, 171
  Withdrawal of Positive Reinforcement, 142–148, 158–161, 171–172
Defining behavior, 11, 176–177
Demonstration-Imitation procedure, 77–80, 94, 96, 110, 132, 165, 233
Denney, Sarah L., 66, 89
Deprivation, 26–28, 33, 35, 50, 53
Diagnosis, 5–7, 21
Differential reinforcement method, 207–208
Dinitz, S., 240
Discrimination, 43–45
Disculturation, 19–20
Disruptive behaviors in home, 225–227
Dix, Dorothea, 19
Dobson, W. R., 43, 177
Dolan, Nancy, 66
Drabman, R., 236
Durability, 98–99, 122

E

Eating, objectionable patterns of, 220–222

Economy, 101–102
Effectiveness, 97, 130
Engeln, R., 145
Environment, 38, 112–113, 121–122
Erwin, W. J., 213
Evaluation, 11, 22, 31–32, 175, 176, 194–197, 205–210
  differential reinforcement method, 207–208
  multiple-baseline method, 207
  reversal method, 206–207
Extinction procedure, 118, 125, 152–158, 166, 171, 214, 218
  case studies, 155–158, 167–168
  compared to Aversive Stimulation, 159–160
  compared to Withdrawal of Positive Reinforcement, 160–161

F

Fading, 80–84, 132
  case study, 93–94
Fading-in, 81
Fading-out, 80–81
Fairweather, G. W., 239–241, 243
Fears, 15–18
Ferster, C. B., 111, 249
Follow up evaluation, 11, 208
Fordyce, W., 9, 222
Fredlund, Delphie, 116
Freitag, G., 105, 163

G

Gaitz, Charles M., 128
Gambrill, E. D., 32
Gelfand, S., 43, 177
Generalization, 44–45, 97–99, 121–122
Generalized-acquired reinforcers, 53–55, 64, 131
  case study, 57–59
Gericke, O. L., 234
Gillis, R., 236
Goals for behavior modification programs, 24–26, 35, 203–205
Goda, S., 77
Goffman, E., 19
Gold, Vivian J., 163
Goldiamond, I., 87, 99, 121, 246, 248, 251
Goodkin, R., 59
Graphing, 192–194
Groups
  behavior modification programs for, 230–244
    community-based reinforcement programs, 236–242
    token reinforcement programs, 230–235
  teaching health-care behaviors to, 111–112
Guiding, 80–84, 132
  case study, 93–94
Guillon, M. E., 119

H

Hahn, Anne, 66
Hall, R. V., 185, 186, 189, 217–218
Hansen, Marc F., 109
Harris, Florence R., 103, 104
Haughton, E., 167
Hawkins, N., 115
Hawkins, R., 225
Henderson, J. D., 237, 239, 240, 243
Henton, K. R., 217
Holland, C. J., 145
Home, disruptive behaviors in, 225–227
Homme, L. E., 61, 249
Honigfeld, G., 236
Hopkins, B. L., 90
Humaneness, 31
Human problems, differing conceptions of, 1–10
Human relationships, 32, 35–36

I

Incompatible behavior, 162–163
Instructing, 74–77, 79, 96, 132, 165, 233
  case study, 90–92

Intermittent reinforcement, 131
Intermittent schedules, 100–104
Interval recording, 186–189
Intervention, 11, 22, 175, 176 (*see also* Decelerating undesirable behavior; Negative Reinforcement procedure; Positive Reinforcement procedure)
Isaacs, W., 87

J

Jones, Mary C., 16

K

Kanfer, F. H., 246
Karnosh, Louis J., 33
Kassorla, Irene C., 163
Kennedy, Trudy, 57
Kinder, M., 105
Krasner, L., 2, 5, 25, 240
Kris, A., 230

L

Lazarus, A. A., 17
LeBow, M. D., 43, 106, 177, 227
Lehrer, P., 230
Leitenberg, H., 213
LeRoux, Rose, 116
Levitt, E. B., 249
Line graph, conventional, 192–194
Linking, 84–87, 132, 233
  case study, 93–94
Lovaas, O. I., 76, 79, 105, 160, 163, 165
Loynd, Jenni, 216

M

Madsen, C. H., Jr., 46–47
Malott, R. W., 248
Mann, Ronald A., 168
Martin, G. L., 236
Martin, P. L., 8, 30, 202, 211, 231
McDaniel, Martha W., 66, 89
McNeal, S., 115
Meaningfulness, 97–99, 121–123, 130, 132–133
Mehrabian, A., 68
Mereness, Dorothy, 33
Michael, J., 157, 163
Milby, J. B., 219
Miller, H. R., 217
Miller, L. K., 111–112, 236
Miller, O. L., 111–112
Mohr, J. P., 213
Monitoring, 111
Motivation, 32–35
Multiple-baseline method, 207

N

Negative Reinforcement procedure, 40, 118, 124–131, 138, 139, 165
  case study, 128–129
Neutral stimulus, 15, 39
Nurnberger, J. I., 249

O

Objectionable patterns of eating, 220–222
Observer agreement requirement, 176–177
Observing behavior, 178–181
O'Leary, K. D., 177, 236
O'Leary, S., 177
Operants, 13–14, 22, 37–38
Osborne, J. Grayson, 56

P

Pain, chronic, 222–225
Pasamanick, B., 240
Patterson, G. R., 98, 115, 119
Patton, Mary E., 217
Paul, G. L., 237, 239, 240
Pavlov, Ivan Petrovich, 14
Pavlovian conditioning (*see* Respondent conditioning)
Percentage of agreement, 195–197
Perloff, B. F., 76

Perrott, Mary C., 111
Peterson, R. F., 79, 178
Phelps, R., 115
Phillips, Jeanne S., 246
Pinel, Philippe, 19
Positive Reinforcement procedure, 10, 30, 36, 45–124, 138, 139, 145, 162, 165–166, 172–173, 180, 203, 204, 206, 212, 214, 226, 235
  administering, 64–69, 131–133
    consistency, 65
    contingent on behavior, 64–65, 124–125
    immediately, 65–67
    potency, 64
    quantity, 67–68, 99
    sincerity, 68
  communities of reinforcement, 122–123
  durability, 98–99, 122
  economy, 101–102
  generalization, 44–45, 97–99, 121–122
  meaningfulness, 97–99, 121–123, 130, 132–133
  producing behavior, 69–97
    Demonstration-Imitation, 77–80, 94, 96, 110, 132, 165, 233
    Fading, 80–84, 93–94, 132
    Guiding, 80–84, 93–94, 132
    Instructing, 74–77, 79, 90–92, 96, 132, 165, 233
    Linking, 84–87, 93–94, 132, 233
    Shaping, 70–73, 75, 77, 79, 87–90 96, 132, 165, 218–219, 233
  socal reinforcers, 104–106
  tapering, 99–104
  teaching health-care behaviors and behavior modification practices, 107–121
    families, 108, 112–116
    groups, 111–112
    individuals, 116–119
    patients, 109, 119–121
  types of reinforcers, 49–63
    acquired, 50–53
Positive Reinforcement (*cont.*)
  types of reinforcers (*cont.*)
    activity (personalized), 55–57, 61–63
    generalized-acquired, 53–55, 57–59
    primary, 50
  (*see also* Withdrawal of Positive Reinforcement procedure)
Powell, J., 128
Preliminary observation, 178–179
Premack, D., 55
Primary reinforcers, 50,
Psychiatric Nurse as a Behavioral Engineer, The (Ayllon and Michael), 157, 163
Putt, Arlene M., 74

R

Ray, R. S., 98
Raynor, Rosalie, 16
Reading, Sadie, 109–110
Recording behavior, 179–181, 185–198
  frequency of activities, 186
  graphing, 192–194
  interval recording, 186–189
  time sampling, 189–191
Reese, Ellen P., 102, 203, 204
Reinforcement programs
  community-based, 236–242
    therapeutic, 239–242
  token, 20, 242–243
    advantages and disadvantages, 233–234
    general description, 230–233
    individual patient and, 234–235
Reinforcer menu, 61, 131
Reinforcers, 26–29, 33–34
  acquired, 50–53, 131
  activity (personalized), 55–57, 61–63, 131
  generalized-acquired, 53–55, 57–59, 64, 131
  intermittent, 131
  primary, 50
  social, 104–106

Reinforcers (*cont.*)
verbal, 59–61
(*see also* Negative Reinforcement procedure; Positive Reinforcement procedure)
Reinforcing Other Behavior, 162–165, 171
Relaxation, 16, 22
Relevance, 97, 121
Remillet, June, 109–110
Respondent conditioning, 13–16, 22
Respondents, 13–18, 22, 37
Response-Cost, 143–145
Reversal method, 206–207
Reynolds, G. S., 33
Rice, H. K., 66, 89
Risley, T. R., 12, 97, 130, 207
Rubenstein, B., 105

S

Sampen, Sue E., 144
Satiation, 50, 54, 148–152, 171
case study, 150–152
Scarpitti, F. R., 240
Schacter, S., 248
Schaefer, H. H., 8, 30, 189, 190, 202, 211
Schaeffer, B., 76, 105, 165
Schiff, L., 230
Schneider, R., 236
Scoles, P. E., Jr., 237, 239, 240, 243
Self-control, development of, 99, 121, 245–253
Self-sufficiency, lack of, 215–217
Setting-the-occasion effect of stimuli, 40–45
Shaping, 70–73, 75, 77, 79, 96, 132, 165, 218–219, 233
case study, 87–90
Shaw, D. A., 98
Sherman, J. A., 78–79, 81, 234
Sherry, P., 82
Silberman, A., 184
Simmons, J. Q., 105, 160, 165
Skinner, B. F., 245
Sloane, H. N., Jr., 144
Social isolation, 217–220
Social reinforcers, 104–106
Stable baseline, 182–183
Stimuli, 14
accelerating effect of, 39–40
conditional, 15
decelerating effect of, 40
neutral, 15, 39
setting-the-occasion effect of, 40–45
unconditional, 15, 16
Stover, D. O., 9
Stuart, R. B., 4, 6, 126, 247, 249–252
Symptom substitution, 4–5, 21
Systematic desensitization, 17

T

Ta, 166–170, 203
Tapering off reinforcement, 99–104
Target behavior, defined, 38
Tate, B. G., 139
Taylor, Josephine, 128
Td, 166–170, 203
Teaching health-care behaviors and behavior modification practices, 107–121
families, 108, 112–116
groups, 111–112
individuals, 116–119
patients, 109, 119–121
Thomas, E. J., 32
Thomas, J., 87
Thomson, L., 213
Time-Out, 118, 143–145
Time sampling, 189–191
Token reinforcement programs, 20, 230–235, 242–243
advantages and disadvantages, 233–234
general description, 230–233
individual patient and, 234–235
Tokens (*see* Generalized-acquired reinforcers)
Treffry, D., 92
Trombly, Catherine A., 65
Turner, Ruby, 9

U

Ullmann, L. P., 2, 3, 5, 25
Unconditional stimulus, 15, 16

V

Valentine, Lois R., 66
Value judgments, 12–13
Variable interval schedule, 101
Variable ratio schedule, 100–101
Verbal reinforcers, 59–61

W

Wahler, R. G., 103, 177
Watson, J. B., 16
Whaley, D. L., 248
Williams, C. D., 114
Withdrawal of Positive Reinforcement procedure, 142–148, 154, 156, 166, 171, 180, 204, 220, 226, 227
case study, 146–147, 168–170
compared to Aversive Stimulation, 158–159
compared to Extinction, 160–161
Within-hospital treatment practices, 240
Wolf, Montrose M., 12, 97, 122–123, 130, 155, 207
Wolpe, Joseph, 17
Wunderlich, Richard A., 95

Y

Yates, A. J., 5

Z

Zeilberger, Jane, 144